Identity and Health

Experiences of health and illness are fundamental to how we understand ourselves, and the postmodern obsession with body image has made health even more significant in identity formation. The study of objective experiences of health and illness can also provide a challenge to traditional objective medical knowledge and, particularly with current healthcare interest in user involvement, can highlight the need for change in health service provision.

This book explores the interplay between identity and health, private and public, mind and body. Drawing on new material, and using and exploring innovative biographical and narrative methods, it covers a broad range of identities in relation to health and illness, including race, religion, ethnicity, disability, age, body image, sexuality and gender.

Identity and Health will be of great interest to academics, researchers and students of sociology, medical anthropology, health and psychology.

David Kelleher is Reader Emeritus in the Sociology of Health at the London Metropolitan University. **Gerard Leavey** is Assistant Director of Research and Development at Barnet, Enfield and Haringey Mental Health NHS Trust.

The contributors include a practising psychiatrist, a researcher and writer on mental health, the Director of Research at the Health Development Agency (HDA), and well-known sociological academics.

We would like to dedicate this book to our parents
May and Jerry
Maureen and Ben

Identity and Health

Edited by David Kelleher
and Gerard Leavey

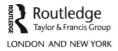

Routledge
Taylor & Francis Group

LONDON AND NEW YORK

First published 2004
by Routledge
11 New Fetter Lane, London EC4P 4EE

Simultaneously published in the USA and Canada
by Routledge
29 West 35th Street, New York, NY 10001

Routledge is an imprint of the Taylor & Francis Group

Typeset in Sabon by Keyword Typesetting Services Ltd
Printed and bound in Great Britain by TJ International Ltd, Padstow, Cornwall

British Library Cataloguing in Publication Data
A catalogue record for this book is available from the British Library

Library of Congress Cataloging in Publication Data
A catalog record has been requested

ISBN 0-415-30791-0 (hbk)
ISBN 0-415-30792-9 (pbk)

Contents

Introduction   vi
GERARD LEAVEY AND DAVID KELLEHER

1. Identity and illness   1
    MICHAEL P. KELLY AND LOUISE M. MILLWARD

2. The meaning of cancer: illness, biography and social identity   19
    SANGEETA CHATTOO AND WAQAR AHMAD

3. Identity and belief within black Pentecostalism: spiritual
    encounters with psychiatry   37
    GERARD LEAVEY

4. Identity and Alzheimer's disease   59
    JANE GARNER

5. The Irish in London: identity and health   78
    DAVID KELLEHER AND GREG CAHILL

6. Sport, health and identity: social and cultural change in
    disorganised capitalism   99
    GRAHAM SCAMBLER, STEFFAN OHLSSON AND KONSTADINA GRIVA

7. Lambegs and bódhrans: religion, identity and health in
    Northern Ireland   123
    RONNIE MOORE

8. Gay and lesbian identities and mental health   149
    MICHAEL KING AND EAMONN MCKEOWN

9. Life narratives, health and identity   170
    MILDRED BLAXTER

Conclusion   200
DAVID KELLEHER AND GERARD LEAVEY

Index   203

Introduction

Gerard Leavey and David Kelleher

'And who are you?', said he. 'Don't puzzle me', said I.
L. Sterne. Tristram Shandy

Within medical sociology, identity has become a significant area of interest, which has brought through the use of phenomenological methodologies the authentic experience of the much-neglected patient into the frame. Kelly and Millward skilfully differentiate between two essential types of identity; an identity that relates to self (private) and an identity that relates to others (public or social). There is of course considerable interplay between the two and it is important to stress that identity is always located in the social. Sociological accounts of identity differ from those found within social psychology in that they tend to focus, respectively, on social experience in the production of identity rather than on internal processes such as personality or cognition. These are not oppositions, as the authors point out, but more the outcome of distinctive disciplinary preoccupations. In order to examine the concept of identity within chronic illness sociological and anthropological perspectives distinguish between disease, essentially a bio-medical concept related to organic pathology and is disconnected to the personal and social dimensions of the individual as they experience illness which is shaped and understood by culture. Given that illness is amenable to cultural influence, it is increasingly understood, if little practised clinically, that the needs and outcomes for patients would be better appreciated and achieved, if attention is paid to the patients' conceptualisation of the problem (Hillier and Kelleher 1996).

For Kelly and Millward (Chapter 1), the importance of medical sociology's examination of identity and illness through the patient experience was not simply that it provided an important conduit for the articulation of suffering, strikingly absent from medical discourse and valuable in its own right, but that it opened up a legitimate and powerful means of challenge to medicine and intensified the need for change within healthcare. Drawing on work within symbolic interactionism such as that of Erving Goffman (1961) the authors view human suffering as not just a 'product of illness' but that it says something more profoundly emanating from the 'the sheer awfulness of the human condition' whereby the essential truth of being human is only grasped through suffering and indeed, redemption through suffering is a motif that runs through much of religious thinking and especially prominent in Judeo-Christian thought on the individual's life journey. In similar vein, at the wider social level it has been suggested that ethnic or group identity is only made transparent when it is in crisis (Mercer 1990). Kelly and Millward, while reinstating the theoretical importance of Parsons' work on the sick role suggest that the concept of identity is an antidote to the flaws in the Parsonian structure in that human experience is brought back into the otherwise rigid prescriptiveness of role (Parsons, 1951). In other words, the patient is not simply a conforming and passive sick object but rather an active participant and manager in the doctor-patient relationship, a relationship that is embedded within a wider social and cultural world – a healthcare system as Kleinman conceptualises it (Kleinman 1980; Kleinman 1978). To some degree, biomedicine has attempted to divorce the body from the person as rational agent, ignoring profound alterations to the self that medical intervention brings. Moreover, the body belongs to the wider community body, acting as both communicative agent and medium. As Lock suggests, the body carries the imprint of the community in terms of habitus, posture, gesture and action (Lock, 1993).

Neither experience nor identity is frozen, fixed in discrete stages but instead they have a malleability that is influenced, but not wholly determined, by social structures. However, while the illness narrative of the patient may provide an articulation of suffering and meaning, the emphasis and reliance on a methodology that is essentially language-based may not have relevance to acute illness. In addition, the construction of meaning through narrative tends to obscure identity change that is embodied and visible. Self and identity gain salience within chronic illness. Thus the body-mind relationship is one of complex mutual influence and one that interacts with the social world. For the individual whose body or bodily function is altered through chronic illness there are correlational changes in the self but contingent upon the extent to which these bodily changes are on view to others (Kelly and Millward 2003a). In the case of young, predominantly female, patients with anorexia nervosa it is argued that bodily change, that is, a natural progression to an identity of sexual maturity is arrested by a determined effort of mind, either conscious or unconscious. Quite literally, the person refuses to grow up and is likely to die in the effort. As with the bodybuilders described by Scambler *et al.* these young people view the body as a project with distorted and ultimately pathologising views of weight, shape and beauty. Likewise, it can be argued that the iconised images of starved beauty generated by a post-modernist obsession with aesthetics and individuality creates a culture where such distortions to perception are inevitable.

Kelly and Millward (Chapter 1) identify four ways in which illness and bodily change in the chronically ill can impact on identity and self. Briefly, these are: the impact on self image rooted in physicality; a conscious regime of maintenance (which in itself reflects the sick identity); a self-consciousness emanating from a 'loss of spontaneity' (Kelleher 1988); and the rupture to previous held conception of self. I can no longer do what I used to, in the same way that I used to do it – am I still the same person? These existentialist questions are developed by Jane Garner.

Kelly and Millward also discuss the link between the personal and social and the way in which the social world assesses, judges and manages deviance by the use of stigma and labelling of individuals and groups who fail to uphold conventions and norms of social etiquette. The difficulty of this labelling for the self is that these responses may become internalised by the individual. By and large, the language commonly employed with respect to people with illness or disability reinforces a conception of the person thus labelled as the illness incarnate – people with severe mental illness become 'schizophrenics'. Goffman's classic work on institutions revealed the 'machinery' of the asylum as it stripped the individual of recognisable (communicated to others and self) instruments of identity and self-hood. Kelly and Millward discuss labelling theory with regard to secondary deviance 'a process of shifting and negotiations that gradually build a deviant self' (Plummer 1979). The authors describe a persistent narrowing of choices faced by the psychiatric patient – setting limits on conduct and reinforcing the identity being conferred. This suppression of self resonates with the views expressed in Leavey's chapter in this book concerning the self-censorship of religious beliefs by young black Pentecostalists with mental health problems who, over time and contact with psychiatric services, come to understand that religious beliefs are often considered as part of the pathology.

Scambler et al. (Chapter 6) consider and challenge universally held assumptions about the salutogenic assumptions that sport is good for you. The challenge is made within the context of globalisation and particularly the transition to disorganised capitalism. They argue that in our post-modernist culture, exercise and sport have become extensions of life-style and consumerist choices. Thus, as illustrated by bodybuilding, the body has become 'the project', 'a site of pleasure and a representation of happiness and success' and where gym culture can be better understood within Foucauldian 'technologies of the self'. The problem however lies in the fact that the pursuit of identity through the glorification of the body, the achievement of 'the look' – the pursuit of an idealised image of youth, fitness and beauty – is unlikely to bring health benefits. In fact bodybuilding is more likely to do harm than good through the use of illicit steroids and excessive bodily strain. Bodybuilding is thus preoccupied by an identity that is visible and external. Sense of self and self-worth is maintained and must be maintained via the body. The authors argue that while post-modernism promises a liberation of sorts for the individual to pursue personal self-constructed identities, the reality is situated more within the highly profitable health and fitness industry and the hypercommodification of global capitalism. The authors examine as the second focus of their challenge, the transition of rugby from a mainly amateur competitive sport to its professional status fired by capitalist need for return on investment ('getting their monies worth'), which in reality means extracting it from the performance of players regardless of risk to health. In addition, the traditional emphasis and veneration of manliness within rugby has, they argue, taken on a harder edge. The nonsense that 'real men' are tough and don't feel pain has cascaded down through male social discourse with huge personal and social costs.

In western societies people are living longer. It should be a cause for celebration but it isn't. Our increasing longevity is presented as a damoclean sword waiting to slice chunks from the public and private purse. The old are not givers, only takers at the social table. To be sure, old age in western societies has rarely achieved the venerated status found within more collectivist cultures but as the preoccupations of post-modernity (beauty, speed, self) bite, the position of older people indeed appears parlous. Old age happens to other people – the young cannot identify with the old. We appear unable to incorporate an image of being elderly into our imagined selves of the future. The importance of continuity as a philosophical concept is one that appears in most discourses on identity, in part because this touches on the existence of a personal, individual human core (in religion sometimes considered as soul) and which has relevance to concerns of ontological security, validity or reliability. Post-modern society characterised by the non-essentialism of rapid change, hybridity, flexibility, identity as consumerist life-style choice and ambiguity undermines the requirement of continuity for identity. With continuity gone, can identity remain? The problem is considered in Garner's chapter on Alzheimers' disease as she discusses the impact of memory loss on dementia sufferers and carers. Can a person exist without consciousness? (Locke 1690). Is memory a complex fiction from which no true identity can emerge (Hume, 1739) or rather, is identity a collection of past selves (Parfit 1971). Philosophically at least, it would appear that identity is understood as unity and continuity ruptured is for the person with dementia. Garner addresses the problem of unity within a humane and pragmatic framework of the person's social context and details of biography and personal values. The implication of continuity within the care of dementia sufferers has a significance that must be considered. If the patient has no memory of being Jewish, religious and married – should we allow these aspects of her 'self' to be also 'buried' by the caregivers? Is identity a sacralised element of humanity and do we violate it through neglect? As Garner points out that, in dementia, although the person has little control over personal identity, the self is not lost.

Western secular notions of identity continue to accept and encompass fragmentation and compartmentalisation of 'self' in a rational and increasingly bureaucratised world, a vision close to that of Weber's disenchanted universe (Weber 1946). Psychiatry as a post-enlightenment discipline has hitched its identity to that of science and, self-consciously perhaps, makes strenuous effort to detach itself from its religious origins. How then should psychiatry address the religious identity and beliefs of people with mental health problems? With a focus on black Pentecostalism in the UK, the fastest growing sector of the religious market, Leavey (Chapter 3) examines aspects of religious identity that are protective to the self-esteem of marginalised or oppressed groups as they encounter the turbulence and anomie associated with modernity and change. Sociological considerations of religion have tended to stress functionalist aspects such as community cohesion and continuity (with perhaps less thought to change and conflict). However, the cognitive, experiential and affective components of religious belief and worship need also to be considered. Pentecostal belief brings unity of identity to the believer or at least attempts to reconcile aspects of the self and its connectedness with the universe. A Pentecostal identity, which is more bound by the spiritual than the material and a belief that healing is always a matter for God, with or without medical intervention is a challenge to a secular psychiatry?

Since the early twentieth century, beginning with studies such as Odergaard's (1932), there is general agreement that contingent upon a number of factors, immigration is linked to higher rates of mental illness (Murphy 1977). Earlier commentators assumed that the explanation lay in the export of psychologically vulnerable individuals. Though the discussion continues, the accepted wisdom suggests that environmental factors related to reception and settlement play a major role. The Irish are often considered the closest migrant group in terms of geography, skin colour, language and a shared troubled history, factors that intuitively might suggest protection. Instead, this largest and oldest migrant group in the UK continues to have the highest rates of severe mental illness (with the exception of schizophrenia), suicide and self-harm for all ethnic and migrant groups. Irish-born migrants in the UK fare no better on physical health. Kelleher and Cahill (Chapter 5) explore the possibility that some of the explanation might lie in the difficulties faced by Irish people as they attempt to maintain an authentic identity (though not always consciously an Irish one), which for a number of reasons fail to achieve value and acceptance. They explore the impact of stereotyping and the destruction of the individual through the imposition of an unwanted collective identity, which is intended to sabotage attempts by the individual to construct or reconstruct a fresh identity. Drawing on recently gathered information through in-depth interviews, Kelleher and Cahill illustrate the diverse range of reasons for migration and the experiences of Irish people in England as their differences collide and the problems this makes in continuing the narrative of identity. The chapter by Moore also uses interview data as a basis for discussing the links between religion, identity and health in Northern Ireland. He illustrates how in Northern Ireland religion forms the basis of culture and cultural differences. He examines how Northern Ireland is a 'region of serious health concerns'. This can partly be explained by poverty and lifestyle but Moore shows the links between religious identity and health, which have not previously been studied. In this chapter the research carried out by him in 1996 for the Department of Health and Social Services is examined in greater detail and used as a starting point for a discussion of the links between religion, identity and health.

Chattoo and Ahmad (Chapter 2), through their research with people facing advanced cancer, attempt an understanding of how such people deal with the disruption to identity caused by the threat of terminal illness. This is made more complex in the context of membership of an imagined moral community (ethnic group). They contend that the intersubjectivity of self comprised of demographic features and connections are not taken for granted truths but have to be constantly negotiated and managed within the progression of illness and treatment and changes occurring to the body. The re-negotiation of identity is seen as particularly difficult in relatively young communities where the experience of cancer is much less common than in the white population. Their mixture of lively narrative accounts balanced with insightful commentary on brief reviews of theoretical literature makes for interesting reading.

Is the construction of a homosexual identity more complex than in other groups such as ethnic minorities or the disabled? Until the latter part of the twentieth century, homosexuality was a diagnosable psychiatric illness and, despite the emergence of a more open, liberal and pluralist society, many lesbian and gay men in Britain face considerable difficulties in achieving an identity not distorted by guilt and shame. King and McKeown (Chapter 8), through their very recent research with lesbian and gay men with mental health problems, examine the encounter between these women and men and psychiatric services. The authors explore a world where heterosexuality is assumed. They examine the impact of these assumptions and how the suppression of a key narrative aspect of identity has a negative impact on mental health.

Blaxter's chapter is also based on narrative accounts which show how identity is constructed, and how 'identity is shown as a grid through which health and illness are perceived and given meaning'. What is also of interest in this chapter is the well-informed discussion of 'story-telling conventions and the purpose of narrative accounts'. The discussion of the theoretical approaches of Frank, Denzin and Bury are used to generate what becomes a comprehensive review of the literature on narrative. This is then used to frame an analysis of her own data, examining how in the thirty-five narrative accounts of her sample past, present and future are inextricably linked in the construction of identity.

References

Goffman E. (1963) *Stigma. Notes on the Management of Spoiled Identity*, Harmondsworth, Middlesex: Penguin Books.

Hillier S. and Kelleher D. (1996) 'Considering culture, ethnicity and the politics of Health' in D. Kelleher and S. Hillier (1996) *Researching Cultural Differences in Health*, London, Routledge.

Hume D. (1739) 'A treatise of human nature', Section VI, 300–12 in D.G.C. Macnabb (ed.) *Personal Identity and Health*, Glasgow, Fontana/Collins; London, Routledge.

Kleinman A., Eisenberg L., and Good B. (1978) 'Culture, illness, and care: Clinical lessons from anthropologic and cross-cultural research', *Annals of Internal Medicine*, 88, 251–8.

Kleinman A.M. (1980) *Patients and healers in the context of culture*, Berkely, CA, University of California Press.

Lock M. (1993) 'Cultivating the body: anthropology and epistemologies of bodily practice and knowledge', *Annual Review of Anthropology*, 22: 133–5.

Locke J. (1690) 'An essay concerning human understanding', Chapter XXVI, 206–20 in A.D. Woosley (ed.) (1964) *Identity and Diversity*, Glasgow, William Collins/Fontana.

Mercer K. (1990) 'Welcome to the jungle' in J. Rutherford (ed.) *Identity, community culture, difference*, London, Lawrence and Wishart.

Murphy H.B.M. (1977) 'Migration, culture and mental health', *Psychological Medicine*, 7, 677–84.

Odegaard O. (1932) 'Emigration and Insanity', *Acta Psychiatrica et Neurologica*, Supp. 4.

Parfit D. (1971) 'Personal identity', *Philosophical Review*, 80, 3–27.

Parsons T. (1951) *The Social System*, London, Routledge and Kegan Paul.

Plummer K. (1979) 'Misunderstanding labelling perspectives' in D. Downes and P. Rock (eds) *Deviant Interpretations*, Oxford, Oxford University Press.

Weber M. (1946) from H.H. Gerth and C. Wright Mills (translated and edited), from Max Weber *Essays in Sociology*, 129–56, New York, Oxford University Press.

Identity and illness

Michael P. Kelly and Louise M. Millward

Introduction

This chapter examines the concept of identity with particular reference to illness. In sociological terms, identity relates to a host of criteria that are called in to play in interaction when assessing oneself and others. It is multi-faceted and has been described in relation to almost every aspect of knowing about oneself and others. Sociologically, identity is understood through visible aspects of the person and all the various points of reference that these might entail, such as skin colour, height, weight, attractiveness, blemishes, deportment, accent and dress attire, for example. It is also understood in relation to abstract ideas, like those that designate communal arrangements, such as status, roles and an almost endless number of group affiliations, such as gender, religion and culture. Conceptually, the term 'identity' consists of two essential types: one regarding others and the assessment of others and one regarding self and the assessment of self. To distinguish these forms the terms 'social or public identity' and 'personal identity or self' are often used.

The development and definition of the concept of identity

It is undoubtedly the case that the idea of identity has exerted a very significant influence on the sociological study of illness and especially chronic disease. By and large, writers dealing with identity have worked within a micro-sociological framework with a focus on interaction. Identity has become a dominant motif within certain strands of medical sociology, especially in Britain. In particular, the study of illness and identity has come to represent an approach to the analysis of ill health in which writers have sought to present the 'authentic' experience of sufferers and give voice to that experience. Because of a commitment to authenticity, phenomenologically and subjectively informed methodologies have been pre-eminent. There is a very rich vein of material dealing with a variety of diseases such as arthritis, diabetes, Parkinsonism and colitis, for example (Anderson and Bury 1988).

The concept of identity has its roots in psychology. However, contemporary social psychology and its concerns with identity have had very little influence in medical sociology. The ways in which sociologists tend to use the term belongs to much older psychological and philosophical literature that has its intellectual origins in the work of William James, John Dewey, Charles Horton Cooley and George Herbert Mead (Kelly 1992). The dualism in the sociology between public identity and self or private identity is present in the original writings of Mead, James and Cooley, and is found subsequently in the work of Goffman (1969) and Rosenberg (1981) and in many other writers associated with the symbolic interaction perspective in sociology (Rose 1962) or, what has sometimes been called sociological social psychology (Rosenberg and Turner 1981).

It is helpful to delineate the dualism at least analytically (even though not all the authors who use the terms identity and self are careful to maintain the distinction). Public identity describes the way we are known, defined and constructed as social beings in interaction with others, and, private identity or self, is the way we are known, defined or constructed by our selves in interaction. Ball (1972) has helpfully distinguished between ego as known to others (identity) and ego as known to ego (self). While obviously these two aspects of person overlap and reinforce each other, given their common roots in social interaction, they can and do diverge, and in the case of chronic illness, that divergence is very important empirically (Kelly 1992).

The following propositions can be derived from this body of work:

1. individuals interactively emerge under social conditions, whereby in relation to others a sense of self is acquired, which consists of a central 'I' and an interactive 'me' (Szacki 1979:406; Denzin 1992:4);
2. mental life is an accessory, rather than an instrumental force; however interactions form certain customs that nurture the mind (Dewey 1922:155; Szacki 1979: 407–10);
3. 'sympathetic introspection' (Meltzer et al. 1975:10) permits people to imagine how they are seen by others (Cooley 1972); and finally
4. through abstract and reflexive language, self arises as a social object that can be interpreted in much the same way as can other objects, whilst retaining an individualistic 'I' (Szacki 1979:425–30).

'Self' or personal identity is not a physical location, it is a cognitive termini borne upon the private sphere of personal thought and language, privately through personally concealed knowing and being and reflexively through one's own appraisal of oneself as seen by others (Kelly and Dickinson, 1997). Charmaz captures the essence of this when she remarks, 'From a sociological view, the self refers to all those qualities, attributes, values and sentiments, including feelings of moral worth, that a person assumes to be his or her own' (Charmaz 1999). Although it is in a constant state of flux, it has a central core against which new information is assessed. The problem of self is that it has to mediate with that which is socially conferred; that which is termed 'social identity'. Social identity is an individual's identity as perceived by others. Social identity can also be accessed, however, through seeing self as others might see self. The notion of James' 'interactive me' describes this idea. The 'interactive me' is the location of 'social identity', namely ones' identity as perceived by others, however through reflexivity it is also the location of self as perceived by self. Social identity concerns the assignment of shared meanings by others. Shared meanings are evident in Dewey's idea of interactions forming certain customs that nurture the mind. These shared meanings can be configured in numerous ways. They might be positive or negative, fleeting or more grounded, structurally determined or personally defined. The problem of social identity is that it is has the potential to fracture previously held conceptions of self and this can be a real issue in chronic illness.

In summary, what has been referred to as personal identity concerns the self; a private cognitive entity of concealed knowing and being that can reflexively appraise itself as seen by others. What has been referred to as social identity, is the product of others' external assignments, which through appraisal, might be subsumed as part of self. Presentation of self as known to self in socially interactive relations where conferred identities align with self are largely unremarkable. Where, however, an individual is continually subject to alternative modes of information that question the essence of self, self must be reappraised. Avenues of alternative modes of information and reappraisals of self are notable events in individuals who experience chronic illness (Kelly 1992).

The ambiguity that is sometimes found in the literature between the individual and social aspects of the person (between self and identity) tends to get reinforced by another characteristic of this literature, which is the absence of an explicit theorising of social structure. Almost all the work on identity and illness focuses on the human agent and on human agency and not on social systems. Of course society is not denied, but it tends to assume either a kind of residual status in the analysis, important as background, rather than an integral part of the processes described, or as constituted within a micro world of face to face interaction. Consequently the agency structure question remains sociologically under-analysed in the literature on the experience of illness and the construction of identities therein.

Sociological descriptions of identity differ from the mainstream social psychological work in a number of ways. General social psychological accounts of identity range from a focus on the cognitive aspects of identity formation and the ways in which people subjectively come to perceive a mature concept of themselves (Erikson 1968; Marcia 1964, 1966) to the ways in which identity can emerge from socially induced individual differences, marks or persuasions. On a wider group level, aspects of identity have been interpreted in various ways such as using occupational status as an anchor for identity (Laliberte-Rudman 2002). The social psychological material tends to focus on the ways in which perceptions and motivations influence various types of identity (see, for example, Salazar 1998). This literature attempts to describe the concept of identity using a multitude of factors that are examined at numerous levels of analyses (see, for example, Worchel *et al.* 1998; Tesser *et al.* 2000; Côté and Levine 2002), but with principal consideration being given to the examination of personality within the parameters of introversion/extroversion, agreeableness, conscientiousness, emotional stability/neuroticism and openness to experience (Ouellette 1999). The real difference between this and the sociological work is the sociologists' emphases on social experience as the basis of identity, rather than its locatedness within cognitive processes or personality traits. The cognitive processes are not ignored in the sociology, in the sense that human beings are seen as thinking beings, but the nature of social experience as it shapes meaning in interaction leading to identity development is given priority in the analysis. This perhaps reflects disciplinary preoccupations rather than any kind of absolute division (see, for example, Honess and Yardley 1987).

Identity and illness experience

Perhaps the best way to understand and define the unique contribution of sociology to the study of identity is to examine the way in which the ideas about the nature of illness experience, as the driver of identity construction, have evolved. Illness experience as a focus of analysis emerges as a means of articulating a difference, sociologically, between disease and illness (Field 1976). Disease relates to physical organic pathology and a biomedical model that does not encompass social, psychological and behavioural aspects of illness (Fitzpatrick 1984). In contrast, illness 'refers to all the *experiential* aspects of bodily disorder which are shaped by cultural factors governing perception, labelling and explanation of the discomforting experience' (Kleinman *et al.* 1978). The experiential nature of illness often transcends the organic realm of disease. This is evident in, for example, situations where diagnoses are conferred in the absence of symptoms but where experiencing the act of a diagnosis is consequential. Illness can be both historically and culturally variable, as is evident in past and present natural, religious and/or spiritual conceptions of illness. In respect of recent work in the context of cultural differences in health, Hillier and Kelleher (1996) note that, 'people's meanings and needs can be better understood by listening to what they say about their own health' (Hillier and Kelleher 1996). In a similar vein, Kihlstrom and Kihlstrom (1999) suggest that consultations with individuals who experience somatisation could be improved by embracing the self-concept of these individuals (1999:33).

The ways in which illness is understood are important for at least four reasons: First, beliefs about illness shape both individual and group experiences of illness. Second, beliefs about illness influence individual and group responses to symptoms (Fitzpatrick 1984). Third, beliefs and potential responses to illness have epistemological links to the ways in which the world is understood through biological, behavioural/psychological and social/environmental realms of knowledge. For example, illnesses such as coronary heart disease are associated with hypertension and cholesterol levels, smoking and physical inactivity, and socio-economic status and social support, respectively (Anderson 1999). Fourth, the relationship between illness and identity is not one-dimensional. Although both self and identity can influence the ways in which illness is perceived and responded to, illness states themselves, in turn, have consequences for self and identity. Illness has the potential to fracture both previously held self conceptions and the perceptions that others might hold of individuals and this is likely to be particularly salient in forms of prolonged chronic illness, as opposed to fleeting episodes of acute illness.

What is undeniable is that one of the major contributions of medical sociology has been to provide a platform for the sociological articulation of the 'authenticity' of the experience of illness. From some of the earliest work by Strauss and colleagues (1984) to the contributions of Bury (1982), Williams (1984), Pinder (1990) and Kelleher (1988), there is a large amount of descriptive material which documents what it feels like to have a particular condition, what it means in social and personal terms, what the impact is on everyday life and what the implications are for the future and the past. Furthermore, this documentation is done largely via the medium of the accounts of the sufferers themselves. The concept of illness careers and the associated identity constructs have helped to place before professional and lay audiences subjective experiences of chronic illness. The ways in which people change about how they feel about themselves and the ways others feel about them, such as how their identities are mediated by these experiences, are described very precisely.

The importance of this is twofold – publicly and theoretically. The theoretical issues we return to later, but by publicly we mean that this literature has been one of the places where the voice of patient experience could be found and was given a public exposure. Before sociologists began to document these processes in this way, the only genres through which such accounts appeared were autobiography or literature. Both are very powerful as a means of conveying the charge of emotional experience, but the sociology added important analytic discipline and purchase as well as academic legitimation. For some writers, the importance of the sociological endeavour in this regard was simply a way of providing a conduit for the voices of sufferers, which were traditionally unheard within professional discourse. So the task of the sociology was simply to lay before new audiences like carers and doctors the true experience of suffering. In doing so the investigations were a means of drawing to the attention of professionals the true nature of the experience of different conditions, in order to bring about change in professional behaviour and practice. (It might also provide further ammunition in the war of attrition with the medical profession, which certain sociologists have prosecuted for the last several decades.) Whatever the intent, one of the unifying themes was that sufferers and carers could readily recognise the accounts as the *real* experience of *real* people struggling with a personal burden of ill health.

But there is another dimension relating to experience in this literature which is seldom articulated sociologically but which seems to us to be deeply embedded within it. This is a concern to describe human suffering, not just as a product of illness, but also as essential to the human condition. Goffman's work (1961; 1963), for example, is shot through with a concern to explore much of the sheer awfulness of the human condition and this existential angst pervades a good deal of the writing on illness and identity. In many of the narratives of illness experience, illness is a metaphor for the experience of life, and an experience of life which is essentially tragic, but (in the Judeo-Christian tradition) there is a kind of redemption through that experience of suffering. Or in Nietzschian vein, the literature contains the Dionysian notion that the true essence of what it means to be human can only be known through suffering, in this case, in severe illness (Benedict 1935).

These latter themes more often than not have their clearest exposition in the accounts offered by the sufferers themselves and reported by the sociologists. These sociological reports have tended to report Dionysian accounts as representative of the experience of illness, *not* as representing the nature of the human condition. Interestingly, the fact that sufferers not infrequently invoke ideas in their accounts of their illness that draw upon the great meta narratives of Christianity or Greek mythology, has tended to go unremarked by the sociologists (Kelly and Dickinson 1997). The idea that chronic illness takes people beyond the normal existential limits leading to greater self knowledge and hence exerting fundamental effects on identity, rings out loud and clear in the patient accounts in the literature. The sociological implications of this, however, are seldom explored. The Nietzschian possibility that the true nature of being is revealed and a deeper self-understanding acquired through illness, tends not to be taken very seriously, even though the voices of the sufferers suggest that it should be.

Theoretically and empirically the importance of identity lies in its critical role in introducing subjectivity into discussions about illness in the face of the dominance of the sick role paradigm established by Parsons (1951). In fact, we would argue that Parsons' depiction of the sick role, for all its detractors, is one of the most significant and important pieces of theorising about the social nature of illness of the last century. His idea that sickness was a form of social as well as biological deviance, that societies developed very precise mechanisms to manage the deviance, and that in the case of modern western industrial societies, these mechanisms took very specific forms and patterned very well defined behaviours, were immensely important. It demonstrated the social as well as the biomedical dimensions of illness and it laid out an agenda for much of the subsequent sociological work on illness.

The concept of illness identity develops, it seems to us, in direct response to several of the perceived inadequacies of the Parsonian system. Identity establishes the primacy of human subjectivity and human agency in the face of the determinism of the social system or of social roles. The concept of identity, as against the concept of role, acknowledges the importance of human agency and interaction in structuring human interaction and leads us away from the apparently prescriptive nature of the Parsonian principles. Identity also acknowledges, especially with its connectedness to the nature of career, the evolving nature of the relationships between doctors and patients which the Parsonian principles tend to under emphasise or at least rather tend to leave in the background of the analysis.

However, above all else, we suggest that the real distinguishing feature of the sociological contribution to the study of illness using the concept of identity, was to give a new sharpness and to illuminate that with which we as lay members of society were already familiar. The ability of sociology to render that which is at once recognisably familiar and yet to shed new light on it, has been a major contribution. Some of the key papers, especially those appearing in the journal *Sociology of Health and Illness*, have done precisely that. So the emphasis on identity in this genre in medical sociology might be conceptualised as a response to Parsons or an elaboration of certain things within the Parsonian framework requiring more attention, especially chronic conditions. In an important sense the idea of identity goes hand in hand with Parsons in establishing an important *raison d'être* for the social, as distinct from the biomedical, in respect of understanding illness. But it also goes beyond Parsons in highlighting the familiar but also profound experience of human suffering, which many illnesses engender.

The processes whereby the social became part of the analysis was however not immediate, even in the wake of Parsons, and the application of the idea of identity played an important role in foregrounding the social. So initially the idea was that disease had social, psychological and economic consequences. (Visotsky *et al.* 1961; Shontz 1975; Albrecht 1976; Platt 1979). In public health circles, the idea that an episode of illness might have economic precursors such as poverty or poor housing was also widely acknowledged (Acheson and Hagard 1984). However, the idea that social and psychological factors were not merely contextual and background residual epiphenomena, but were an integral part of the being, meaning, causes, consequences and experience of illness, owes its debt to Parsons. Identity theory applied to illness by sociologists provided the explanation of the ways in which such things could be theorised and drew out the essential self reflexive nature of the experience of illness and its significance to the wider human condition.

The conceptual journey is in itself quite informative. Two papers, which have charted the history of the way sociologists have dealt with illness experience and identity, are those by Lawton (2003) and Pierret (2003). In reviews of articles in *Sociology of Health and Illness*, over a twenty-five year period, they provide a narrative of the way these ideas have evolved. What these two authors describe is the gradual broadening of interest by sociologists in their concerns about identity and the experience of illness. The interest expands from simple descriptions of the experience as a set of stages operating in chronological sequence, to a concern to illuminate the meaning of experience. In other words, the idea of *chronos*, of linear sequential time, gives way to the idea of *kairos*, concerned with the fusion of past, present and future in biographical significance. The idea that experience is more than the chronicle of a series of events is displaced by the notion that experience is socially located and constructed, on the basis of interpretation and understanding, and that events can come to have different meanings in retrospect and in prospect. The idea that identity simply moves through a series of discrete stages or progressions is replaced by the idea that identity is malleable and plastic and bounded by social structures but not determined by them. Bury's seminal paper (1982) on biographical disruption perhaps best exemplifies this position. A couple of years later, Williams' paper on the linguistic accounting processes which accompany biographical disruption and repair (1984) moved the focus of the analysis still further from time sequences towards an understanding of the language of the sufferers of illness and the subtle nuances which language brings to bear on the experience and its retrospective and prospective understanding.

Subsequently, the question has arisen as to whether the discovery of these linguistic elements of story telling or narratives of illness is little more than a methodological artefact rather than the core of identity. In other words the identification of processes which are fundamentally linguistic are identified as the product of a methodology – the use of in depth interviewing – which requires subjects to produce accounts about themselves, with themselves at the centre of the narrative. As new evidence emerges it also becomes clear that a focus on chronic illness as against acute illness leads to an overemphasis on issues of disruption and biography, and that acute illness and indeed some forms of chronic illness do not share these kinds of characteristics. The most interesting development though has been the recognition that an over emphasis on language and the construction of meaning can in turn lead to a description in which the body and bodily processes are overlooked. The fact that the management of bodies that do not function in the way that people either want or which society deems to be age and gender appropriate, is at the heart of the experience of illness and the construction of public identity (Kelly and Field 1996). Changes to the body are at the centre of visible changes in identity and the way people feel about themselves. So a stream of literature, which has explored the relationship between the body and identity in illness, has also emerged (Millward and Kelly 2003a). This in its turn has led to the development of the idea that the material and physical world should be reintegrated into the understanding of identity (Lawton 2003; Pierret 2003; Kelly 2001).

Illness, identity and the biological and social world

In chronic illness, self and identity gain salience. It is the biological realm of the physical body that prompts this process. The physicality of the body is important for self and identity because it is inextricably associated with self and with identity. Whilst an essential link between the body and self and identity relates to the body's capacity for cognitive thought, the body is important for self and identity in a number of other respects. Bodily characteristics are part of what individuals perceive themselves to be and influence the ways in which cognitive thought by self and by others are configured. Bodily characteristics are relative to private and public perceptions in relation to both the aesthetic physicality of bodies and the functioning physicality of bodies (Kelly 1992); categories that are not entirely mutually exclusive. Private personas of self and others' perceptions of individuals are constructed upon a range of aesthetic bodily qualities, such as being attractive, ugly, tall, short, fat, thin and such like, and a range of functional bodily qualities which span both capacities of physical functioning such as being able to run, jump, reach, climb, and capacities of cognitive functioning, such as the ability to learn, to remember, or to recognise. The crux of the relationship between the body and identity is that where there are chronic alterations in the aesthetics and/or functions of the body, the self that is configured upon that body must also change. The potential for an altered identity, however, is contingent upon the nature of the bodily changes and whether these come to be subject to public gaze (Millward and Kelly 2003a). These ideas are highlighted in various patient accounts. For example, for subjects who had had ulcerative colitis cured by major surgery, the experience of bodily pain, changes in bodily symmetry, the addition of a 'new body part' and profound changes to sanitation routines resulted in compulsory permanent changes in both private conceptions of self and in tensions arising between the choices of revelation and secrecy in public management and presentation of self (Kelly 1992). For these subjects, appliances were not only a private matter, the permanent demands of attaining and mastering secrecy and the potential for exposure were located in the social world (Kelly 1992). Similarly, individuals with diabetes, a metabolic condition, have experienced, or are at risk of experiencing, a range of physical bodily changes such as impaired vision, infected wounds, tiredness and impotence (Kelleher 1988).

For these individuals, the chronically ill physical body was associated with self and identity in at least four ways:

- because the impact of physical bodily changes altered the image that individuals had of themselves;
- because to maintain physical equilibrium and prevent further physical risk sequelae, the physicality of the body itself required a special and unique form of physical maintenance not required by majority groups;
- because the routines of managing the body impinged upon previously routinised ways, a recurrent theme that Kelleher referred to as 'loss of spontaneity' (Kelleher 1988); and finally
- because the chronically ill physical body had the potential to invoke extended meanings that assaulted and ruptured a previously held conception of self.

A common thread between both of these groups of individuals and others who have chronic illnesses is the way in which public spheres of life become the site of intense negotiation with huge implications for self and identity. In public spheres the self not only seeks social legitimation, acceptance and integration, but does so equipped with stocks of shared knowledge about the kinds of conduct that are necessary for these events to occur. Bodies that 'malfunction' deviate from norms in both a private and public sense. Public management, however, concerns the social world and the attribution of identity. In the social world it is not just the physicality of the body that has to be managed; far more overwhelming and difficult to influence, predict and control are the cognitive appraisals of others in relation to presentation of self and yet these also have to be managed.

Whilst the previous paragraphs noted how the salience of self and identity in chronic illness is prompted by the biological realm of the physical body, this section notes how the salience of self and identity in chronic illness can be maintained by the social realm of interaction. The social world is where the generation of meanings has profound consequences for self and identity. The social world judges the physical and cognitive presentation of individuals in relation to cultural conventions, and shortcomings are defined by the societal standards therein. The links between illness and identity are illuminated in the social world largely because chronic illnesses and their maintenance have the potential to deviate from social standards. This deviation has the potential to occur within the ways that society is structurally configured and within societal configurations of individual agency. In both of these realms, society manages this deviance by the use of stigma and labelling techniques.

Labelling is a reaction to groups and/or individuals who, through chronic illness, cannot uphold the networks of physical and cognitive behaviours that social etiquette demands. The problem of this labelling for self is that these labels have the potential to become internalised.

One of the key ways in which illness links to identity is through the legitimation of a medical condition by a member of the medical profession. This legitimation might be sought after or undesirably imposed. In both cases the professionally conferred identity is drawn from a recognised classification of disease states that bears consequences for the ways in which particular illnesses and their severity are afforded different statuses and the ways in which these might lead to such things as access to additional resources. Often overlooked, however, are the ways in which medical professionals also invoke a range of other identities and themselves engage in stereotypical processing.

Goffman (1961) highlighted how psychiatric professionals required the removal of individuals' clothing and its replacement with hospital attire and discouraged any references to their personal life. At the same time encouraged adaptation to their new location. This stripped individuals of their very essence of self and avowed a hospitalised patient identity. The importance of this for patients with mental illness was that the resulting patient behaviour reinforced their identity as a mentally ill patient. These links between illness and identity are described in Lemert's (1951) primary and secondary deviance thesis. Primary deviance concerns changes in self that are induced from minimal tensions between self and the environment. In primary deviance, self is largely unaltered. Secondary deviance concerns profound changes in self that are induced through a progressive process of tensions between self and environment. Plummer described secondary deviance as 'a process of shifting and negotiations that gradually build a deviant self' (1979:105). The key issue in secondary deviance is that persistent narrowing of choices, as for example being a mental patient, sets limits on conduct. This unwittingly reinforces the identity being conferred. Secondary deviance is where individuals adopt a socially conferred identity as part of self and come to behave in ways that are associated with their new self.

The notion of the Parsonian sick role discussed earlier (Parsons 1951) offers another idea of how medical professionals can invoke a range of alternative identities and engage in avowing stereotypical identities onto patients. In brief, a patient's occupation of the sick role is legitimated by doctors who, for temporary illness states, and as long as individuals pursue the goal of recovery, grant these individuals exception from their normal social duties. Because, however, chronic illness is not a temporary illness state, legitimation of illness and the rights and obligations therein are not always warranted by the sick role. Sociologically, this is an important event because patients who do not fit a 'legitimate patient identity', and therefore the sick role, often fail to legitimate the doctor's own role in the encounter. It is, in other words, sociologically not very neat. Doctors have to manage not only the often-continued presence of the chronically ill patient, but also the possibility of their own role being called into question. What is at stake is that some patients deny the role of the professional (Kelly and May 1982:154) and the issue of problem patient becomes bound up with professional identity (May and Kelly 1982:292). The method by which doctors respond to this dilemma is through the use of labelling as, for example, is exemplified in the notion of 'heartsink patients'. Patients become associated with a host of stereotypical labels such as demanding, uncooperative and manipulative; qualities that are not necessarily inherent in the patient; rather they are qualities that, through frustration and defeat, the doctor comes to assign to the patient (Millward and Kelly 2003b). These labels are a situational response to a therapeutic dilemma that concerns the nature of the doctor's role and where, within the doctor-patient encounter, that role is not legitimated (Millward and Kelly 2003b). In doctor encounters, social etiquette demands that the patient fulfils a number of socially defined criteria and failure to do so heightens the potential for labelling. These labels confer an identity on to the chronically ill patient. An identity that the patient is often aware of.

Charmaz (1999) provides a critique of the sick role in this context, arguing that its application does not highlight essential links between illness and identity. For Charmaz, the sick role fails to acknowledge that recovery is not always possible; it assumes a lack of culpability for illness that does not account for the stigma and blame that can attach to illness; it provides exemption from social roles whereas chronically ill individuals might opt to preserve roles, and it assumes a hierarchical doctor-patient relationship, whereas chronic management can involve shared information and decision making. The problem, for Charmaz, is that, 'An abstract role analysis fails to account for subjective experience and its meaning for patients' (1999:230). What Charmaz fails to note, however, is that it is difficult to expect any one role to cover the full spectrum of subjective experience and meaning for patients. Individuals occupy several roles simultaneously and although one role might be salient at a particular moment in time, illness identities are configured using numerous roles and numerous phenomena.

The links between illness, identity and human agency are bound up in day-to-day social interactions and their meanings are rendered precarious by the various physical and/or cognitive limits that chronic illness invokes. These limits are subjective in the sense that they are relative to the pre-illness self. In chronic illness, the numerous personal identities that constitute self and the socially induced meanings that attach to these identities, such as what it means to be male, a mother, a teacher, an employee and so on, are disrupted. Bury (1982) used the term 'biographical disruption' to describe how chronic illnesses induce a profound disturbance of the taken-for-granted aspects of everyday life that straddles cognitive and material modes of thought and mobilises concerns about uncertainties, resources and lay and professional modes of thought (Bury 1982). In biographical disruption, it is difficult for self to remain intact.

Focusing on a sample of chronically ill males, Charmaz (1994) describes how the biographical disruption of illness induces dilemmas for self and identity. She notes the ways in which self consists of several personal identities, which for men, link to social networks of meanings that are bound up with masculinity, such as male athlete, the competitive businessman and the 'Viet Nam' veteran. Other identities, however, related to age, being a husband and so on. These identities are part of self and in chronic illness, are forcibly reassessed. For example, for heart attack or stroke patients, relatively simple everyday events, such as bathing and grooming, now had to be mastered; a situation that threatened their masculinity. Illness can also set limits on some identities, such as those that are tied to the labour market (Lalibert-Rudman 2002). People can also use illness identities as a reasoning strategy. For example, in Charmaz's (1994) study identities tied to the life-cycle were used to explain away illness as a mid-life crisis. In this respect, illness prompted the links between self and the ageing process; a process that has its own identity formations (Coleman 1996).

In illness, identities can unwittingly become reaffirmed. For example, Charmaz (1994) found that the identity of chronically ill married men was reinforced by the attention, comfort and care of their wives and families. This also reinforced their status within the household and their links with the pre-illness self, a feature not evident in the accounts of single men. On the other hand, an identity could become denied. Where individuals lost hope of influencing the degenerative course of illness and cognitively separated the illness from mainstream life, and thus from self, significant others could sometimes refuse to engage in this 'bracketing' (Charmaz 1994).

A problem of chronic illness for self and identity is the extent to which human agency can keep illness concealed by successfully accomplishing covering and passing. Scambler and Hopkins' (1985) subjects accomplished 'passing' by citing alternative reasons to epilepsy to account for why they could not drive; 'covering' was accomplished by referring to minor seizures as 'fainting fits'. In Charmaz's study one subject did not attend swim or cocktail parties in order to conceal his restricted diet and dialysis shunt (Charmaz 1994). Linked to passing and covering is the idea of 'information control', whereby parents of children with epilepsy did not use the term epilepsy outside the home environment to prevent the child's awareness of the social connotations of the term (Scambler and Hopkins 1985).

Visibility is a key feature for identity markers, which typically becomes a master status and a master identity. 'It is master status because this position overrides and subsumes others; it is a master identity because it defines every other identity' (Charmaz 1994:48). Even where physical or cognitive impairments are not visible, 'felt stigma' (Scambler and Hopkins 1985) can subtly transmit social identity. 'Felt stigma' is more pervasive than 'actual' stigma because it is generated through shared meaning and renders individuals on constant guard.

In some circumstances an illness identity is readily accepted because of the secondary gains that it entails. On a basic level, these gains can include enhanced caring and attention of others and access to resources, such as financial or more suitable housing. Acceptance of an illness identity can also help individuals to accomplish successful social relationships. Scambler, for example (1991:190) notes Higgins' (1980) converse notion of avoidance, whereby individuals with hearing impairments extended their 'stigmatised' attribute by also acting mute as this permitted them to rely on the written word which eased social relationships.

Identity dilemmas described above appraise self in relation to past, present and future in a combination of ways. Armstrong and colleagues (1998), for example, describe how the process of genetic counselling which provides patients with a genetic identity, that in contrast to other identities, is an old one that is newly revealed; an identity that is reconstructed in the past as well as in the future. In contrast, Orona (1990) describes how Alzheimer's disease involves a loss of identity that results in a self that resides only in the current. In Alzheimer's the ability to recall past selves is lost, an event that also prevents the individual validating the identity of others.

A range of personal identities is tied to the very core of self. These identities are laden with social meanings. Chronic illness questions the claim to these identities. In males, for example, 'With each identity loss from chronic illness, preserving valued past "masculine" identities becomes more difficult' (Charmaz 1994:52). There are some suggestions that the impact of illness symptoms are evaluated in relation to their impact on the identities that individuals consider to be more salient, rather than in relation to pre-existing knowledge about illness representation (Levine and Reicher 1996; Levine 1999). This is an interesting point as it helps to indicate some of the ways in which individuals might refute a particular identity. For example, a study of disabled individuals found that the vast majority did not accept a disabled identity because impairment was not considered an important aspect of their sense of self or personal identity (Watson 2002). The crucial matter here is the extent to which individuals can successfully incorporate or challenge socially induced identities and where this is not possible, the extent to which individual agency can accomplish minimising or concealing techniques that forestall or prevent negatively attributed identities.

Conclusion

This chapter has appraised the links between illness and identity using the sociological concepts of self and identity in relation to biological and social modes of being. The relationship between illness and identity is not uni-linear; it is multiplex and relates to biological, social and physical worlds. In chronic illness, the self-persona, its presentation and public negotiation merge with these worlds through bodily attributions, socially structured institutions, 'doing' routines of daily interaction and through the resources of the material world. This idea captures the ways in which these worlds are saturated with identities. For 'normals', these identities often have a dormant quality. For individuals who experience chronic illness, however, their dormant status becomes volatile and their potential to actively impact on the lives of sufferers is intensified.

Previous attempts to understand the experiences of chronic illnesses, including the impact of deviant identities and statuses have used particular notions of an illness career (see, for example, Goffman 1961; Fabrega and Manning 1972). For Goffman, the term 'career' was bound up with the concept of institutionalisation and how experiences of hospitalisation, for example, strip individuals of a self. For Fabrega and Manning (1972), 'A career implies a potential beginning, intervening stages with distinctive properties, and equally important, an end' (1972:103). Whilst the career model of illness has been useful for gaining insight into a range of illness-related phenomena, illness identities do not reside solely in chronological time as implied by these models. Illness identities are constant features of biological, social and physical modes of being. They are malleable and constant, they exist in linear time and in social experience constructed and reconstructed in language and interaction. They develop out of experience and the constituent public and private identities, identity and self, themselves interact and evolve. The experience of illness, especially chronic illness, tends to exert a force that separates self and identity empirically as well as analytically. In understanding the tension between self and identity we are able to get a view of the experience of illness which captures the finer nuances of that experience and which helps to reveal the elemental nature of the biological, social and physical modes of suffering and say something quite profound about the very nature of human existence itself.

References

Acheson D. and Hagard S. (1984) *Health Society and medicine: An Introduction to Community Medicine*, third edition, Oxford, Blackwell.

Albrecht G. (1976) 'Socialization and the Disability Process' in G. Albrecht *The Sociology of Disability and Rehabilitation*, Pittsburg, University of Pittsburg Press.

Anderson N.B. (1999) Foreword in R.J. Contrada and R.D. Ashmore (eds) *Self, Social Identity and Physical Health*, Oxford, Oxford University Press.

Anderson R. and Bury M. (1988) Living with Chronic Illness: The Experience of Patients and their families, London, Hyman.

Armstrong D., Michie S. and Marteau T. (1998) 'Revealed identity: A study of the process of genetic counselling', *Social, Science and Medicine*, 47, 11, 1653–8.

Ball D. (1972) 'Self and Identity in the context of deviance: the case of criminal abortion' in R.A. Scott and J.D. Douglas (eds) *Theoretical Perspectives on Deviance*, New York, Basic Books.

Benedict R. (1935) *Patterns of Culture*, London, Routledge and Kegan Paul.

Bury M. (1982) 'Chronic illness as biographical disruption', *Sociology of Health and Illness*, 4:167–82.

Charmaz K. (1994) 'Identity dilemmas of chronically ill men', *The Sociological Quarterly*, 35, 2, 269–88, reprinted in A. Strauss and J.M. Corbin (eds) (1997) *Grounded theory in practice*, London, Sage Publications.

Charmaz K. (1999) 'From the "Sick Role" to stories of self', in R.J. Contrada and R.D. Ashmore (eds) *Self, Social Identity and Physical Health*, Oxford, Oxford University Press.

Coleman P.G. (1996) 'Identity management in later life' in R.T. Woods (ed.) (1996) *Handbook of the Clinical Psychology of Ageing*, London, John Wiley and Sons Ltd.

Cooley C.H. (1972) 'Looking-glass self' in J.G. Mannis and B.N. Meltzer (eds) *A Reader in Social Psychology*, 2nd ed. Boston, Allyn and Bacon Inc.

Côté J.E. and Levine C.G. (2002) *Identity, Formation, Agency and Culture: A Social Psychological Synthesis*, New Jersey, Lawrence Erlbaum Associates.

Denzin N. (1992) *Symbolic Interactionism and Cultural Studies: The Politics of Interpretation*, Oxford, Blackwell Publishers.

Dewey J. (1922) 'Communication, individual and society' in J.G. Mannis and B.N. Meltzer (eds) *A Reader in Social Pychology*, 2nd ed. Boston, Allyn and Bacon Inc.

Erikson E.H. (1968) *Identity, Youth and Crisis*, New York, Norton.

Fabrega H. and Manning P. (1972) 'Disease, illness and deviant careers' in R.A. Scott and J.D. Douglas (eds) *Theoretical Perspectives on Deviance*, New York, Basic Books Inc., 93–116.

Field D. (1976) 'The social definition of illness' in D. Tuckett (ed.) *An Introduction to Medical Sociology*, London, Tavistock.

Fitzpatrick R. (1984) 'Lay concepts of illness' in R. Fitzpatrick, J. Hinton, S. Newman, G. Scambler and J. Thompson (eds) *The Experience of Illness*, London, Tavistock.

Goffman E. (1961) *Asylums*, Harmondsworth, Middlesex, Penguin Books.

Goffman E. (1963) *Stigma. Notes on the Management of Spoiled Identity*, Harmondsworth, Middlesex, Penguin Books.

Goffman E. (1969) *The Presentation of Self in Everyday Life*, Harmondsworth, Middlesex, Penguin Books.

Higgins P. (1980) *Outsiders in a hearing world: A Sociology of Deafness*, Beverley Hills: Sage.

Hillier S. and Kelleher D. (1996) 'Considering culture, ethnicity and the politics of health' in D. Kelleher and S. Hillier (eds) *Researching Cultural Differences in Health*. London, Routledge.

Honess T. and Yardley K. (1987) (eds) *Self and Identity: Perspectives Across the Lifespan*, London, Routledge and Kegan Paul.

Kelleher D. (1988) 'Coming to terms with diabetes: Coping strategies and non-compliance' in R. Anderson and M. Bury (eds) *Living with Chronic Illness: The Experience of Patients and their Families*, London, Unwin Hyman.

Kelly M.P. (1992) 'Self, identity and radical surgery' *Sociology of Health and Illness*, 14: 390–415.

Kelly M.P. (2001) 'Disability and community: A sociological approach' in G.L. Albrecht, K.D. Seelman and M. Bury (eds) *Handbook of Disability Studies*, Sage, London, 396–411.

Kelly M.P. and Dickinson H. (1997) 'The narrative self in autobiographical accounts of Illness', *Sociological Review*, 45: 254–78.

Kelly M.P. and Field D. (1996) 'Medical sociology, chronic illness and the body', *Sociology of Health and Illness*, 18:241–57.

Kelly M.P. and May D. (1982) 'Good and bad patients: a review of the literature and a theoretical critique', *Journal of Advanced Nursing* 7, 147–56.

Kihlstrom J.F. and Kihlstrom L.C. (1999) 'Self, sickness somatization, and systems of care' in R.J. Contrada and R.D. Ashmore (eds) *Self, Social Identity and Physical Health*. Oxford, Oxford University Press.

Kleinman A., Eisenberg L., and Good B. (1978) 'Culture, illness, and care: Clinical lessons from anthropologic and cross-cultural research', *Annals of Internal Medicine*, 88, 251–8.

Laliberte-Rudman D. (2002) 'Linking occupation and identity: Lessons learnt through qualitative exploration', *Journal of Occupational Science*, Vol. 9, No. 1, 12–19.

Lawton J. (2003) 'Lay experiences of health and illness: past research and future agendas', *Sociology of Health and Illness*, 25 Silver Anniversary Issue: 23–40.

Lemert E. (1951) *Social Pathology*, London, McGraw-Hill Book Co. Inc.

Levine R.M. (1999) 'Identity and illness: The effects of identity salience and frame of reference on evaluation of illness and injury', *British Journal of Health Psychology*, 4, 63–80.

Levine R.M. and Reicher S.D. (1996) 'Making sense of symptoms: Self-categorization and the meaning of illness and injury', *British Journal of Social Psychology*, 35, 245–56.

Marcia J.E. (1964) *Determination and Construct Validation of Ego Identity Status*, unpublished doctoral dissertation, Ohio State University, Columbus, OH.

Marcia J.E. (1966) 'Development and validation of ego identity status', *Journal of Personality and Social Psychology*, 3, 551–8.

May D. and Kelly M.P. (1982) 'Chancers, pests and poor wee souls: problems of legitimation in psychiatric nursing', *Sociology of Health and Illness* 4, 279–301.

Meltzer B.N., Petras J.W. and Reynolds L.T. (1975) *Symbolic interactionism: Genesis, varieties and criticism*, London, Routledge and Kegan Paul.

Millward L.M. and Kelly M.P. (2003a) 'Incorporating the biological: Chronic illness, bodies, selves, and the material world' in S. Williams, L. Birke and G. Bendelow (eds) *Debating Biology: Sociological Reflections on Health, Medicine and Society*, London, Routledge.

Millward L.M. and Kelly M.P. (2003b) 'Doctors' perceptions of their patients' in R. Jones, N. Britten, L. Culpepper, D.A. Gass, R. Grol, D. Mant and C. Silagy (eds) *Oxford textbook of primary care*, vol. 1, Oxford, Oxford University Press.

Orona C.J. (1990) 'Temporality and identity loss due to Alzheimer's disease', *Social, Science and Medicine*, 10, 1247–56, reprinted in A. Strauss and J.M. Corbin (eds) (1997) *Grounded Theory in Practice*, London, Sage Publications.

Ouellette S.C. (1999) 'The relationship between personality and health: What self and identity have to do with it' in R.J. Contrada and R.D. Ashmore (eds) *Self, Social Identity and Physical Health*, Oxford, Oxford University Press.

Parsons T. (1951) *The Social System*, London, Routledge and Kegan Paul.

Pierret J. (2003) 'The illness experience: state of knowledge and perspectives for research', *Sociology of Health and Illness*, 25: Silver Anniversary Issue: 4–22.

Pinder R. (1990) *The Management of Chronic Illness: Patient and Doctor Perspectives in Parkinson's Disease*, London, Macmillan.

Platt S. (1979) 'The impact of chronic illness on the family with special reference to mental handicap' in M. McCarthy and P. Millard (eds) *Management of Chronic Illness*, London, King Edward's Fund for London.

Plummer K. (1979) 'Misunderstanding labelling perspectives' in D. Downes and P. Rock (eds) *Deviant Interpretations*, Oxford, Martin Robertson, 85–121.

Rose A.M. (1962) (ed) *Human Behavior and Social Process: An Interactionist Approach*, London, Routledge and Kegan Paul.

Rosenberg M. (1981) 'The self concept: social product and social force' in M. Rosenberg and R. Turner (eds) *Social Psychology: Sociological Perspectives*, New York, Basic Books.

Rosenberg M. and Turner R. (1981) (eds) *Social Psychology: Sociological Perspectives*, New York, Basic Books.

Salazar J.M. (1998) 'Social identity and national identity' in S. Worchel, J.F Morales, D. Páez and J.C. Deschamps *Social Identity: International Perspectives*, London, Sage Publications.

Scambler G. (1991) 'Deviance, sick role and stigma' in G. Scambler (ed.) *Sociology as Applied to Medicine*, 3rd ed., London, Baillière Tindall, 185–96.

Scambler G. and Hopkins A. (1985) 'Being epileptic: coming to terms with stigma' in U. Gerhardt and N. Wadsworth (eds) *Stress and Stigma*, London, Macmillan, 26–43.

Shontz (1975) *The Psychological Aspects of Physical Illness and Disability*, New York, Macmillan.

Strauss A., Corbin J., Fagerhaugh S., Glaser B., Maines D., Suczec B., Wiener C. (1984) *Chronic Illness and the Quality of Life*, 2nd ed., St Louis, Mosby.

Szacki J. (1979) *History of Sociological Thought*, London, Aldwych Press Ltd.

Tesser A., Felson R.B. and Suls J.M. (2000) *Psychological Perspectives on Self and Identity*, Washington, DC, American Psychological Association.

Visotsky H., Hamburg D., Goss M. and Lebovits B. (1961) 'Coping behaviors under extreme stress: observations of patients with severe poliomyelitis', *Archives of General Psychiatry*, 5: 423–8.

Watson N. (2002) 'Well, I know this is going to sound very strange to you, but I don't see myself as a disabled person: identity and disability', *Disability and Society*, 17: 509–27.

Williams G. (1984) 'The genesis of chronic illness: narrative reconstruction', *Sociology of Health and Illness*, 6: 97–104.

Worchel S., Morales J.F., Páez D. and Deschamps J.C. (1998) *Social Identity: International perspectives*, London, Sage Publications.

2

The meaning of cancer: illness, biography and social identity

Sangeeta Chattoo and Waqar Ahmad

Theoretical background

This chapter is an attempt to understand the narrative reconstitution of self for people facing advanced cancer, especially when the bodily integrity of self is threatened by terminal illness, marking the self as discontinuous and fractured. We then go on to explore how legitimacy of certain forms of practical strategies and symbolic styles (cf. Bury 2001) might be central to restoration of self and identity, enabling people to 'keep a narrative going' (cf. Giddens 1991) despite biographical discontinuities and disruptions. We also explain how claims to membership of an imagined moral community such as an ethnic group, often perceived as a well defined whole, might be fragile and rest on contested meanings and values underpinning illness narratives that are shaped by a complex interplay of biographical features of ethnicity, gender, age and socio-economic position. It is our contention that intersubjectivity of self, that cuts across ethnic, gender, age and class affiliations, is negotiated differently in relation to the uncertain and changing nature of the illness and treatment. Hence, both temporality and biographical context are central to how identities are threatened and/or maintained in the face of a life threatening illness.

We take the example of advanced cancer since it brings into sharp relief the notion of self as discontinuous at various levels, and how continuity is forged through particular narratives informed by larger discourses and collective representations to sustain particular identities. Our biographical approach (see Radley 1993; Williams 2000:53) can potentially address how a particular appropriation of an illness narrative might provide a critique of existing relationships and biographical circumstances, moving between the existential, inter-subjective, the cultural as well as structural dimensions of the illness (and caring) experience.

It is important, at this point, to reiterate the specificity of advanced cancer as a disease category before we move on to specific issues of illness and identity. Cancer shares much with other illnesses characterised by chronic, acute as well as terminal features where temporality is marked by uncertainty, fear about recurrence or spread, and a dialectic between hope and despair. The metaphoric associations between cancer and a painful, lingering death, however, mark it as a prognostic disease (Sontag 1991; Stacey 1997). The diagnosis and treatment of cancer is an emotionally loaded process for the patient, family and friends as well as the professionals (Luker *et al.* 1995; Stacey 1997; Yates and Stetz 1999; Schou and Hewison 1999). Apart from the implications of the diagnosis itself, people often face loss of a part of the body, temporary or permanent loss of function as a consequence of surgery, chemotherapy, radiotherapy or hormonal treatment. Not only is there often a lack of overlap between symptoms and signs here, but also the boundaries between curable and incurable, and treatment and palliation are fuzzy and often left undefined by the professionals – something Schou and Hewison (1999) describe as a minimisation strategy.

The shift from curable to palliative treatment is pre-empted as the logical, natural progression of the disease and, hence, a continuity within the discourses and practices of oncology and palliative care (two major specialities dealing with cancer). However, the person who is ill often experiences these events diachronically, as a series of apparently disconnected events unfolding in time within a pre-existing biographical context. This results in discontinuity created by a focus on prognosis, uncertainty about treatment outcomes and the notion of time that takes on a new meaning, compromised ability to plan for future in relation to commitments, and the ability to take care of one's own self.

Needless to say, cancer, like other chronic and life-threatening conditions, raises the issue of meaning at two levels (see Bury 1982). At one level are issues related to practical, physical *consequences* of the symptoms and impending impairment and uncertainty that can cause disruptions in everyday routine at home and/or at work. At another, closely related level, are issues related to practical, physical *significance* of the symptoms that can have serious consequences for a person's identity. These impinge upon deep cultural, symbolic values related to cancer that might carry a historically and culturally specific stigma based on variance from a perceived norm for gender/age related body image; ideas related to health and lifestyle; impairment or and disfigurement; ideas related to ageing and so on.

We might, at this point, reflect on Sontag's (1991) unsuccessful but evocative plea for disassociating the metaphoric and moral connotations from the experience of cancer as an illness. Contrary to her vision, better scientific knowledge and the endeavours of medicine at controlling the disease have not succeeded in demystifying the metaphors and stigma of a 'spoiled identity' for people suffering from cancer. There is no way of living and dealing with cancer outside the meaning ascribed to the illness within a particular culture (see, for example, Stacey 1997). Orr (1993, as in Fosket 2000: 20–1), in response to the Foucauldian notion of disease as defined by the social and political imperatives of a particular biomedical discourse, has suggested that illness is more than the summation of the biomedical features of the disease and cannot be reduced to the power of the clinical gaze. It refers to the '... particular relations to the scene in which it materialises as a form, a cultural, economic, symbolic and gendered scene that includes, but is never restricted to the site of medical practices'.

It is important to acknowledge that feminist theory, especially as applied to the sociology of knowledge, has led to a sophisticated understanding of the subjugation of experiential and subjective knowledge of women in relation to chronic illness. For example, Fosket's work (2000) on women's construction and experience of breast cancer shows how the dominant mode of biomedical knowledge, and power legitimised through it, simultaneously constitutes a contesting site for competing knowledges related to personal, embodied as well as shared experiences. It seems to us that this understanding of competing knowledges has wider significance and can be applied to the experiences of women as well as men suffering from different kinds of cancer, or other serious conditions. However, the site of competing knowledge and legitimate understandings of the illness might have multiple foci, not only within but also outside the clinical setting – within the family, kin network or the community. Further, we suggest that reducing medical knowledge to power and control excludes alternate understandings of medicine as a system of healing within which the dimension of power co-exists with faith in the doctor or the healer.

We argue that narrative reconstructions of self in the face of a life threatening illness need to be seen as part of a critique of self, significant others and society. Seale (1998:30) has suggested that these narratives often project self and significant others as morally right, and just, even when the bonds are being threatened by breach of norms or expectations thereby '... maintaining the legitimacy of the speaker's claim to membership of an imagined moral community'. We shall see how the imagined moral community itself might be a sight of contesting values and conflicting perceptions of self in illness.

Methodological note

Since our approach relies on contextual interpretation of the narratives (cf. Bury 2001 below) of people who are ill themselves or closely involved in caring for someone, a note on the notion of narrative and the narrative method would seem appropriate. One characteristic feature of narrative is that the story changes with unfolding events – 'maintaining several provisional readings' of the past, present and future, potential plots based on available social scripts (Good 1994:144). Hence the story is never finished in most cases, addressing the contingent in life with the *subjunctive* mood or open possibility, incorporating memory and desire (Good 1994:146); often highlighting conflicts in interpersonal and social life through gaps and silences within the narrative account.

Having set the wider theoretical and methodological scene, the rest of the chapter addresses the meaning of cancer and social identity by drawing on empirical accounts of people and their experience of cancer. The data presented here was collected as part of a larger qualitative study looking at the needs and experience of South Asian and White patients, and their main carers, in relation to advanced cancer (see Chattoo *et al.* 2002). A purposive sample of 56 South Asian (Indian, Pakistani and Bangladeshi origin) and 19 White people between the ages of 19–85 years of age who were suffering from advanced (metastatic) cancer, but well enough to take part in the research, was drawn through contacts with oncology, palliative care and hospice teams from across Leeds, Bradford and Leicester. We used in-depth interviews with 54 patients and 41 carers/close family members or friends to understand their engagement with illness, treatment and interface with health professionals across statutory and voluntary sectors of care, supported by contextual information gathered through formal and informal interviews and observation with various professionals, a patient self-support group, and community members.

The analysis relied heavily on a biographical approach (see Chamberlayne and King 2000:18), contextualising different narratives on illness and caring within a family, and comparing these across families and ethnic groups to understand the salience of ethnicity in relation to gender, age and socio-economic position in shaping the illness and caring experience of the research participants. While our analysis draws similarities and differences between the experiences of the ethnic groups, we avoid reducing individual experience and explanations to generalisations made for the collective. The following section provides an overview of this interface between the shared experience of cancer within an ethnic group and biography, followed by a section on narrative reconstitution of identity, focusing on gender and ethnicity, in relation to various losses suffered by an individual due to cancer, and threats to the notion of a competent self, highlighting the intersubjective context within which narratives are generated, legitimated or silenced. The names of participants appearing hereafter have been anonymised.

The interface between biography and collective representations of cancer

We have argued elsewhere that the collective experience of cancer is informed by the epidemiological features of the disease, and the history and demography of a particular (ethnic) community (see Chattoo *et al.* 2002), informing the collective representations or the symbolic and cultural values associated with cancer. Thus, the shared experiences of White families in relation to cancer are, to a large extent, located within an ageing society where every third person is affected by cancer, whilst cancer accounts for a quarter of all deaths. Clinically, the disease is associated with ageing since two-third of cancers are diagnosed in people over 65 years of age. Comparatively, the overall relative mortality from cancer of the common sites as compared to the White population is significantly lower within the South Asian populations that have a younger age profile. Nevertheless, cancer accounts for approximately one in six deaths among South Asians and, therefore, is an important cause of morbidity and mortality within these communities (Barker and Baker, 1990; Winter *et al.* 1999), and is expected to increase as the cohort of middle-aged Asians grows older (see Bahl 1996; Coleman and Salt 1996).

It is not surprising that irrespective of striking similarities in the experiences of patients and carers from across the range of ethnic groups, there are significant differences related to the demographic features of the communities and shared experiences and collective memory of cancer. A majority of the White participants had some experience of seeing or caring for a relative or friend with cancer, and had some idea about the role of professionals and services involved in palliative care. At the same time, the image of a close relative or friend suffering impairments, premature ageing, or dying a lingering, painful death pre-empted their own future and imminent death as well as their interaction with particular professionals. This comes out strongly in the following excerpt from Melissa Brown's interview. Melissa was 55, a secretary by profession, and suffered from fibrous histocytoma resulting in extensive thigh surgery and loss of mobility. She had been closely involved in taking care of her aunts in the past, and did not wish her son, grandchildren and the rest of the family to have to care for her.

> I don't know, looking back how it was when we were nursing my three aunts. It's not a place for little children to be in because that would leave them awful memories ... If I wasn't going to get well, I wouldn't want them see me past a certain point. I'd like them to see me when I'm still Nana ... I remember when the Macmillan nurse came to my aunt at the night ... to give her morphine ... she said to my granddad, 'How is your wife tonight?', because my aunt, who was his daughter and about thirty years younger, looked as old as my granddad! She looked so horrific and my other aunt did (too).

Further, the metaphoric association between cancer, ageing and a painful, lingering death shaped the attitudes of White participants towards hospices that were perceived as a dying space, and the Macmillan nurses as representing the 'old and the dying'. This response is well represented in the voice of one of the younger patients, Kate Shaw, a 26-year-old woman of working-class background, who had a five-year-old son, and was suffering from advanced melanoma. Kate knew her prognosis but when offered a

Macmillan nurse, she resisted, 'I am not having a Macmillan nurse. I don't need one ... they are for the old and the dying'. As well as symbolising a social and public acceptance of one's terminal status, the Macmillan nurse also embodied the fear and stigma associated with cancer in the wider culture (see also, Small and Rhodes 2000:71). In contrast, a majority of the South Asian families reflected fragmented family histories with people spread across continents at various points of time, with little personal experience of a close relative with cancer, associated services and professionals in the field, or hospices.

Another interesting difference between the White and the South Asian experiences related to the manner in which many older South Asian participants subsumed their cancer within the larger category of chronic health problems and losses associated with old age. Old age in this case serves as a rhetorical device for understanding the randomness of the disease and individual suffering, which does not necessarily resolve the ontological issues related to pain or facing imminent death. Ikhlaq Din Mir, an 80-year-old man of Pakistani origin with a history of assorted working-class/middle-class jobs, had prostate cancer that had spread to his spine and was painful and incapacitating. Reflecting on his unexpected recovery from a serious drug reaction during his recent stay at the hospice where he was admitted for pain control, he commented, 'It is only up to Allah – for how long he wants to keep me here. *I am in old age* – who knows how long I have to live? It is all up to him' (our emphasis).

Here, Ikhlaq Din notes both the significance of old age and the will of Allah to account for an affliction which otherwise may be difficult to under-stand. However, Ikhlaq Din's reference to Allah must not be equated with fatalistic despondence since the notion of 'Allah's will' is often complementary to the notion of a duty to feel responsible and seek treatment (see Chattoo 1990; Atkin and Ahmad 2000).

In contrast, a majority of the older White patients held old age at the periphery rather than the centre of their illness narrative. In fact, Harry Johnson, a 70-year-old retired teacher, felt offended when the interviewer queried whether he thought his prostate cancer might be seen as part of the normal process of ageing itself:

> ... my brother, the one who is very helpful to me, I don't think he was quite so helpful at that time because he attributed it (symptoms) to old age and nothing else. And I said to him, 'It's not old age. I'm ill, I know I'm ill'. ... and he said, 'Harry, we are all getting older', and I couldn't get past that and I stopped discussing the subject with him.

In fact, Harry believed that if the GP had not missed his diagnosis, he would still have around 10 to 15 years of a healthy life to live. It might be suggested that Harry's disregard for the link between ageing and certain types of cancer reflects the larger cultural framework surrounding health and illness within which old age is treated as obsolete within Western cultures, a problem beyond the scope of this discussion. In contrast to Harry, the narratives of the younger White as well as South Asian patients (especially those between 19–35 years of age), with one exception, constructed cancer as the disease of old age. The association of cancer with the old and the dying resulted in a lack of contemporaneity with other (older) cancer patients and a feeling of not belonging with them, especially on the oncology wards – described by a young woman patient attempting black humour as the 'death row'. This is well represented by Ahsan Ahmad, a 29-year-old man of Pakistani origin, who had been unemployed since he was diagnosed with cancer of the stomach that had spread to his liver:

> Obviously it does affect you, when I was on . . . the cancer ward, I was the only young person. Everybody else was old and you feel very strange that other people are ill in their older age and they've enjoyed life but I am having these experiences at this age . . .

Within this construction of cancer, age is significant to how the illness is experienced and shared with others, whilst marking the (younger) self as different from the 'old and the dying' constitutes an important mode of discursive consciousness in order to survive and maintain hope in a seemingly hopeless situation.

Against the backdrop of the wider context outlined above, the following sections draw on individual experiences of people suffering from advanced cancer, focusing on the role of gender and ethnicity, bringing to life the intersubjectivity of self experienced as *discontinuous* within the context of a life threatening illness. We use this space to explore how the notion of a discontinuous self addresses both context and content (meaning) of particular losses related to life threatening illness, and disruptions to bonds and commitments – so central to one's identity – as well as aspects of reinforcement of self-identity in the face of serious illness. Our focus on gender and ethnicity is not to minimise the impact of socio-economic position and, within the context of minority communities, its conflation with the notion of ethnicity, or the centrality of (biographical rather than chronological) age, alluded to earlier, in shaping the illness experience. Also, our focus on women's narrative is a conscious theoretical choice to sustain the argument in relation to gender and particular losses related to cancer.

We assume that '. . . ethnicity is as much the product of internal arguments of identity and contestation as of external objectification' (Werbner 1997: 18), thus being contingent and situational. Our focus is on understanding how, at an individual level, particular markers of identity such as ethnicity and gender, rather than being innate attributes of a group, become salient within a particular context of negotiation, contested claims to the meaning of illness and identity, and reaffirmation of a competent self in relation to significant others. Our aim here is to suggest one theoretical frame within which the complexity of the interface between markers of identity and life threatening illness can be analysed without relegating the experience of ethnic minority people to a separate, second hand or subaltern speciality of 'ethnicity', a common mode of exclusion within mainstream sociological research.

Negotiating the contingent boundaries of self and identity

In this section we analyse how bodily integrity, that we assume to be central to a notion of competent self across cultures (Giddens 1991), is threatened by the experience of cancer, and how these threats are experienced and negotiated by women, in relation to particular biographical features. One of the significant features of cancer is that, apart from the implications of a particular diagnosis itself, people often have to face loss of body part, and temporary or permanent loss of function as a consequence of surgery, chemotherapy, radiotherapy or hormonal treatment. People, including small children, associate sudden loss of hair with cancer. Loss of hair, there-fore, is seen as marking the self apart as a cancer sufferer, a *stigmata*, making 'passing' as normal or as having other chronic, less threatening conditions difficult (Stacey 1997; and Goffman 1963 on passing in general). This can be especially problematic for some of the South Asian patients who might not wish to share details about the illness within their community due to various imperatives discussed elsewhere (see Chattoo *et al.* 2002). Some try to protect elderly parents or children, especially if they live overseas, whilst others want to protect their own identity and therefore want to keep the news of the illness within close family. Further, whilst loss of hair following chemotherapy can be difficult for men, a majority of White as well as South Asian women in our sample found it particularly difficult since both texture of hair and hairstyle were perceived as markers of their femininity and individuality.

Loss of appetite, weight loss (or weight gain associated with hormonal treatment) and tiredness are often experienced as an index of a disintegrat-ing embodied self, causing great emotional distress to the person who is ill as well as significant others. The emphasis on food and eating, for example, apart from highlighting the nature of significant relationships and any breaches thereof, symbolises an inherent struggle to survive, marking the self as discontinuous (see also Seale 1998:149–71). Some of this is reflected by Jean Blake, who was 64 years old and suffering from cerebral metastasis secondary to breast cancer which had spread to her arm and her leg. She had severe lymph oedema and had lost much of the function of her right arm and hand despite recent surgery and an ongoing course of (palliative) chemotherapy. Jean lived on her own, and although she was well supported by her elder daughter, sons, and a close friend and neighbour, as her illness worsened, she was finding it increasingly difficult to eat and take care of the routine:

> Um ... and I'm not eating and I've dropped a stone. I'm very upset about it but I know why I dropped it. Um ... so as I say, I had ... my friend brought me some chicken in a sauce yesterday, and I ate about what? About three, three dessertspoons is all I managed, because I'd been retching as well. I've been very retchy recently, and a lot of it is nerves as well, you know? Um ... but I ate half of that yesterday, and then just half a sandwich ... I don't know why? But I've not done bad, and I feel all right. You just feel as if you've had a six-course meal, you know ... Um ... , I get very tired quickly. I'm quite depressed, because nothing's working quickly. And then my eyesight started going about six weeks ago ...

It is important to note here that Jean's depression was polysemic, representing different aspects of her life within which loss of appetite, loss of energy (tiredness) and other losses related to the illness were contextualised. At one level, Jean was referring to the physical and psychological impact of her cerebral metastasis. She had lost function of her right arm following surgery (and was learning to write with her left hand at the time of the interview). She wasn't able to drive her much loved jeep parked outside and missed packing her grandchildren off to a quiet picnic in the greens, and doing her own shopping whenever she pleased. She was losing her sight and found it difficult to carry on with the routine. Jean was undergoing (palliative) chemotherapy at the time, which meant dealing with nausea, loss of appetite and loss of strength so that she could barely drag herself out of bed on 'bad' days. She observed that instead of getting better with the various treatments, as she had expected, she was 'going down' and 'losing parts' of herself.

At another level, Jean's narrative focused on disruptions caused by her illness affecting her roles as a single woman, a mother and a grandmother desperately trying to maintain her independence at home, seeking minimal help from family, friends and professionals. Most significantly, Jean was still coming to terms with the fact that she had to send her disabled (younger) daughter, Katie, into residential care who was an integral part of her self and every day life. She suddenly realised, '... that I would not be able to look after her again. Um ... so that was another heartbreak that sent me down again. I was heartbroken, you know, so that didn't do me any good ...'.

Jean's narrative highlighted the significance of temporality and the biographical context within which she defined and experienced 'losing parts of herself'. Faced with a life-threatening illness that was taking away parts of her self, the story of her breast cancer (diagnosed three decades ago) and mastectomy belonged to a past, discontinuous from the present. However, for a majority of other women irrespective of their ethnicity and, to a large extent, their age, mastectomy had specific implications for their gendered identity due to its polyvalence in relation to the notion of a 'whole' body, as well as notions of womanhood.

As observed by Hallowell (2000:173–174) with reference to women's narratives on prophylactic mastectomies, '... bodily identity and integrity is important for their sense of self-identity, in so far as the body parts implicated in this instance – the breasts – were constructed as internally related to gender identity'. A majority of the women in our research shared a sense of grief in relation to mastectomy, though a few (irrespective of age) constructed it primarily as a worthwhile bargain for survival. Sukhbir Singh, who was in her fifties, equated loss of breast with loss of a gendered identity itself, 'It leaves you in the abyss – neither here (woman) nor there (man) – like a *hijda* (eunuch)!' The significance of the discontinuity posed by mastectomy goes beyond the notion of disfigurement that reconstruction is expected to address. It incorporates a notion of 'materiality of the body', so well described by Hallowell (2000), as well as a notion of the body as a whole (see, for example, Chattoo 1990). It is hardly surprising that Sitara Rehman, who was 50 at the time, was still able to recollect the numbness and shock that she felt 18 years ago when a (male) doctor suggested that she would have to have her breast removed – inspiring her to subvert the male, medical authority:

> ... I goes, 'what?' He says, 'nobody will notice the difference'. I don't know what else he was saying. He must have been saying other things that I wasn't hearing. And that was it. It was like somebody had poked me with a needle and I jumped up two feet. I said, 'If somebody took your thingamajig out and filled your underpants with plastic? ...'

The notion of body as a whole in relation to mastectomy leads us to the link between gender, ethnicity and membership of a moral (religious) community, and its implications for the construction of self as discontinuous. We explain the link through the narrative of Hasina Ullah. The narrative reconstruction of her illness takes us through the *significance* of cancer and mastectomy in relation to self, significant others as well as community on one hand, and the shift from being curable to being terminal on the other. It reveals how temporality and the changing symbolic context of cancer and its treatment are implied in the practical strategies for sharing information within family, and negotiating ruptures caused for the self. Finally, we suggest that Hasina seeks an alternate closure to her story of a life unfulfilled and coming to an end through a shift of discursive consciousness towards a religious script. This shift, we suggest lends narrative continuity, making her suffering meaningful.

Gender and ethnicity in negotiating loss of breast

Hasina Ullah was a 34-year-old Muslim woman born in Bangladesh but brought up in England. Hasina lived in a mixed, lower-middle-class neighbourhood with her husband who worked as a financial advisor, and two daughters and a son between the ages of 12 and 15. She had been working as a factory supervisor. She had always been an independent woman with a car of her own, who enjoyed working and doing childish things with her children that their father did not much care for. All that changed when things started to go wrong and Hasina was diagnosed with breast cancer.

Hasina had no particular knowledge about breast cancer, its symptoms and their implications since nobody among her family or friends had cancer. She had been experiencing frequent pain in the shoulder that she attributed to work related stress and for which she eventually visited her GP who prescribed some painkillers. The pain persisted and she had an X-ray that did not reveal anything significant. Later on she had pain in her armpit for which her GP prescribed her more painkillers without examining her. Retrospectively, Hasina was upset at what she described as her GP's 'negligence' and the lack of co-ordination within the healthcare system.

One day Hasina noticed that her nipple was inverted; she knew something was seriously wrong. Hasina was initially reluctant at the idea of a male doctor examining her but eventually she was examined and referred to hospital for a biopsy. It took over two years for Hasina to have a diagnosis. The doctor at the hospital explained the disease and that she needed to have her breast removed, emphasising that her chances of surviving without surgery were bleak. Initially Hasina refused to consider mastectomy as her only option since it threatened her sense of being a woman, and she was worried about the impact it might have on her relationship with her husband:

> … I was afraid. I want(ed) to look nice in front of my husband … you know. I felt it's not nice without a breast but he didn't care. He said, you know, 'I want you to get better'.… So he said, 'I don't care how you look like. I just want you to live'.… I used to think in my mind, you know, what he's going to think …

Hasina's husband persuaded her to believe that she needed to undergo the operation for his sake and that of their children. Hence, like many other women across ethnic groups, Hasina constructed her trauma of losing a breast as an extension of her obligations towards her husband and her children; preserving her identity as a carer and 'a self-in-relation' (cf. Hallowell 2000:173–4).

At the hospital, the breast care nurse had tried to address Hasina's concern about loss of breast by showing her pictures of other women who had a prosthesis, reassuring her that her loss would not be visible to others.

Clearly, Hasina's concerns related to the bodily integrity and *materiality* of her body in relation to her gendered identity (cf. Hallowell 2000) that could not be contained within or restored by the idea of prosthesis. It was her notion of the 'body as a whole' that was being threatened and nobody, except her husband, was to share that sense of loss. Furthermore, loss of breast also posed a threat to her claim to membership of her (Bengali-Muslim) ethnic community, creating another rupture and source of discontinuity in her narrative. Her narrative reveals how her claim to membership remained fragile, resting on contested symbolic meanings and values associated with her loss, whilst the community appears as disablist and repressive rather than nurturing and supportive – a contesting site for moral constructions of self and suffering (see also Hussain *et al.* 2002). What is important is that in her discursive consciousness, Hasina attempts a subversion of the authority of this symbolic-moral collective by redefining the boundaries between the conjugal, kin and social relationships within her narrative. This demanded an entirely different practical strategy to 'keep her narrative going', as we explain below.

Claims to membership of her own ethnic community, however, were far from secure and put a lot more at stake, as is clear by the practical strategy deployed by the couple to maintain her identity within the Bengali community. Hasina and her husband decided not to disclose the diagnosis to the children at that time. Choosing the right time and space to disclose such emotionally sensitive information to small and vulnerable children is a common strategy adopted by parents across ethnic groups (see Chattoo *et al.* 2002; Lawton 2000). The children were told that their mother was having surgery and treatment for shoulder pain. They also decided not to disclose the diagnosis and the details about the surgery to Hasina's natal family, her parents in-law (who lived in Bangladesh) or anyone else within the extended family.

Despite Hasina's emotional proximity to her mother who was closely involved in her care during and after the surgery, even her mother was not told about the mastectomy. One of the reasons for concealing details was to protect her mother from the painful news itself and the other was to protect her own identity within the Bengali-Muslim community. Hasina did not wish to burden her mother since she felt that, '. . . it would hurt her more to keep it inside' since it was likely that she would share the bad news with other members of the family, and that the news would spill out within the community (a common concern within South Asian communities across religious and cultural divide). The couple feared that people within the community might ask awkward questions and ridicule her for her loss of breast. It is important to caution here that although there are no obvious religious reasons surrounding this construction of loss of breast within Islam, the explanations for illness and such loss might be constructed differently at an experiential level, within the broader context of meaning of suffering. Hence, whilst the biomedical definition and understanding of her illness created an alternate and competing understanding of her loss and experience in Hasina's own narrative, the cultural construction of this loss was simultaneously located within a contesting site of moral values and definition of self.

Clearly, the moral 'community' (analytically *not* synonymous with a religious ideology) appears here as a conflicting site of construction of self and illness that the act of silence and secrecy seems to subvert, whilst claims to legitimacy within it remain problematic. However, such secrecy was tedious and achieved at an emotional price. In fact, in a mood of desperation, Hasina had said to her husband, '... well I even thought about that, if I die then people will know obviously (through rituals of bathing and preparing the body for burial). And then my husband said, "Well, that is going to be different, you won't be there ..."' What is further important is that the spread of the disease is treated almost as a separate category, as we saw in Jean's case, and the moral reverberations for self are constituted differently in relation to significant others.

Loss of independence and reverberations for self

Following surgery and chemotherapy, Hasina believed that she was recovering until she woke up one morning and heard one of her breast-bones crack. The pain was excruciating. She was lying in bed and couldn't get up:

> ... same breast, well the bone, yeah, and then my husband ran up stairs and he saw me sitting on the floor. I couldn't get up and this is where I felt tears in my eyes because ... I didn't cry, all these things happened, you know, like chemotherapy and operation, I didn't cry. And that day I cried a lot ...

Further on:

> I couldn't even walk to the bathroom and I thought to myself, 'what is going on', you know? ... after all the operation and the chemotherapy I *knew* (believed) I am going to gain something – I will be better. And that day I knew I couldn't walk. ... and I thought, 'How am I going to do my things, you know, wash myself, having bath? I don't want to ask my husband ....

The possibility of loss of physical mobility and independence posed a different kind of threat to Hasina's integrity of self. As emphasised by Giddens (1991:57), bodily discipline is intrinsic to the competent social agent across cultures. Complete and constant bodily competence is central to communication, social interaction and to maintenance of ontological security. We need to locate this major shift in Hasina's discursive consciousness within the sequence of events related to her illness; the sudden threat of loss of independence in relation to personal care brought on by the spread of the disease subsequently marking her status as 'palliative'.

At the time of the interview, Hasina was coming to terms with the fact that she was 'seriously ill' and did not have long to live. There were days when she couldn't get out of bed and she was upset that her house looked neglected since she wasn't able to take care of routine household chores. This was a concern she shared with a majority of other women who perceived a neglected or 'dirty' house as a sign of a failing self. It might be mentioned in passing that, like other women across ethnic groups, she had declined the offer of home help – treating it as an infringement of privacy and a sign of a failing self. One of the recurrent themes in Hasina's narrative relates to how she drew moral boundaries around selfhood and caring, even though she had an ideal, caring husband, loving children and a family who were happy to help:

> I don't want to give trouble to my mum you know, she is my mum after all, she would be happy to help you but still I don't want to give anybody trouble. For example, making a cup of tea, I don't feel like telling my children. I want to do it myself and sometimes I can't do it and I start crying you know. This is horrible and I thought to myself if I live as long as ... I can do it myself ... *if I can't do things myself then I don't want to live* ... (our emphasis)

Later on she added, 'yes, I feel some kind of half human, who can't do things, helpless...' As mentioned earlier, she treated her compromised independence as a threat to her ontological status as a human being. The threat incorporated a notion of cultural competence as an ability to sustain identities through important roles and relationships rather than merely choice, autonomy, control and reflexive planning premised on a notion of risk and expert knowledge, as envisaged by Giddens (1991).

On one hand, the knowledge about her prognosis prompted Hasina to come to terms with the possibility of imminent death, loss and grief marking a rupture in her narrative on her 'normal life', hopes and desires and the life she had enjoyed with her family. On the other hand, her narrative turns to alternate explanations for her illness within a discourse that suggests a possible closure, recasting her story by marking her suffering as redemptive. Hasina mentioned that she had been angry with herself (for not recognising the first symptoms) and, at times, with her Allah for what the illness had done to her. However, this is how she explained it to herself:

> If I look at my life, I never had a bad time. I had a very good married life and my childhood was very good ... everybody took care of me. I never

had to suffer for anything in my life ... I used to pray to God, 'Don't give my children any disease. I can't bear to see them suffer. Give it to me and I can take it ...'.

Hence, in 'taking the illness upon herself', an act of redemption, as it were, she was grateful to Allah that her children and family were safe and well, and that apart from this illness, she 'never had a bad time'. We might add that, in seeking an explanation from religion, this possible closure to Hasina's narrative reinforces the inter-subjectivity of self in relation to her illness, making her suffering meaningful by reaffirming her identity as a mother and a wife despite the various discontinuities brought on by her illness, as highlighted in her account earlier. We tried to show how these discontinuities and threats to her identity were addressed and negotiated through parallel, reflexive critiques addressing various dimensions of her life and illness experience.

Conclusion

This chapter highlights the significance of inter-subjectivity in analysing narrative reconstitution of self and identity in relation to cancer as a form of life threatening illness. We have discussed the metaphoric associations of cancer as a prognostic disease and the meaning of various losses associated with this disease at an interface between individual (biographical) and shared experiences of a family within an ethnic community. The case of advanced cancer brought to light the centrality of the notion of discontinuity and fractured self in understanding the impact of cancer on different aspects of identity. We saw how, across ethnic groups, threats to bodily integrity and notions of cultural competence are negotiated as attempts at sustaining significant roles and relationships, rather than independence and autonomy *per se*. Using a biographical approach, we argued that these negotiations involve an interplay between contingent and complex markers of identity such as gender, age, ethnicity or class, and the salience of one or more of these rests on the particular context within which claims to a particular form of identity are being asserted, contested or reaffirmed.

Without belabouring the point, we would like to suggest that the notion of an inter-subjective self that, we assume, cuts across gender, age class and ethnic divisions challenges the notion of a unique, autonomous self responsible for taking moral decisions, implicated in both Giddens's theory as well as dominant Western medico-legal notion of personhood. Further, contingency and inability to plan for future, and discontinuity, often central to the experience of people facing life-threatening illnesses such as cancer, don't fit well with this notion of self premised on autonomy, cultural competence defined as control, choice and reflexive planning (see also Lawton 2000). It also problematises the notion of an authentic voice that can be located within an autonomous patient or a carer, highlighting the intersubjective context within which illness narratives are generated, contextualised, sustained or silenced.

Finally, we hope to have shown that an analysis of narrative reconstitution of self and illness within a comparative framework, in Seale's phrase (1998: 31), goes beyond '... the mythologies of Western individualism and avoids over-romanticised versions of subjectivity'. Hence, we reiterate the need to move away from the tendency towards romanticising and individualising narrative forms premised on a notion of 'authentic selfhood' marked by the experience of pain and suffering (cf. Frank, 1995 and others), and focus on social-structural dimensions of narratives in relation to gender, class, age, race or ethnicity (see also, Williams 2000).

Acknowledgements

Our thanks to the patients and their families for sharing their experiences with us; to the Cancer Research Campaign and the Department of Health for funding the study; our collaborators Rosemary Lennard and Mary Howarth for their unstinting support and healthy criticisms; Mari Lloyd-Williams, Anita Pabla and Liz Penny for their generous help with fieldwork; oncology teams at St James' Hospital, Leeds, especially Geoff Hall, and Bradford Royal Infirmary; Marie Curie Centre and Manorlands (Sue Ryder Home), Bradford; St Gemma's Hospice and Wheatfields hospice, both in Leeds; LOROS, Leicestershire hospice; our advisory committee for their guidance; and colleagues at CRPC for their support, especially Karl Atkin for helpful comments on an earlier draft of the paper.

References

Atkin K. and Ahmad W.I.U. (2000) 'Family caregiving and chronic illness: how parents cope with a child with a sickle cell disorder or thalassaemia', *Health and social care in the community*, 8, 1: 57–69.

Bahl V. (1996) 'Cancer and ethnic minorities: the Department of Health's perspective', *British Journal of Cancer*, 74 (suppl XXIX): 332–40.

Barker R.M. and Baker M.R. (1990) 'Incidence of cancer in Bradford Asians', *Journal of Epidemiology and Community Health*, 44: 125–9.

Bury M.R. (1982) 'Chronic illness as biographical disruption', *Sociology of Health and Illness*, vol. 4, 2: 167–82.

Bury M.R. (2001) 'Illness narratives: fact or fiction?' *Sociology of Health and Illness*, vol. 23, 3: 263–85.

Chamberlayne P. and King A. (2000) *Cultures of Care: Biographies of Carers in Britain and the two Germanies*, Bristol, Policy Press.

Chattoo S. (1990) 'A Sociological Study of Certain Aspects of Disease and Death: A Case Study of Muslims of Kashmir', unpublished thesis, University of Delhi.

Chattoo S.C., Ahmad W.I.U., Haworth M. and Lennard R. (2002) 'South Asian and White Patients with Advanced Cancer: Patients'and Families' Experiences of the Illness and Perceived Needs for Care' (Final Report to CRC UK and The Department of Health), Leeds, Centre for Research in Primary Care, University of Leeds.

Coleman D. and Salt J. (1996) *Ethnicity in the 1991 Census* (vol. 1), London, HMSO.

Fosket J. (2000), 'Problematising biomedicine: Women's constructions of breast cancer knowledge' in L.K. Potts (ed.) *Ideologies of Breast Cancer: Feminist Perspectives*, Basingstoke, Macmillan.

Frank A. (1995) *The Wounded Storyteller: Body, Illness, and Ethics*, Chicago/London, The University of Chicago Press.

Giddens A. (1991) *Modernity and self-Identity: Self and Society in Late Modern Age*, Oxford, Polity Press.

Good B.J. (1994) *Medicine, rationality, and experience: An anthropological perspective,* Cambridge, Cambridge University Press.

Goffman E. (1963) *Stigma: Notes on the Management of Spoilt Identity*, Englewood Cliffs, N.J., Prentice Hall.

Hallowell N. (2000) 'Reconstructing the Body or Reconstructing the Woman? Perceptions of Prophylactic Mastectomy for Hereditary Breast Cancer Risk' in L.K. Potts (ed.) *Ideologies of Breast Cancer: Feminist Perspectives*: 153–80.

Hussain Y., Atkin K. and Ahmad W.I.U. (2002) *South Asian Disabled Young People and their Families*, Bristol, Policy Press.

Lawton J. (2000) *The Dying Process: Patients' experiences of palliative care*, London/New York, Routledge.

Luker K., Beaver K., Leinster S. *et al.* (1995) 'The information needs of women newly diagnosed with breast cancer', *Journal of Advanced Nursing* 22: 134–41.

Orr J. (1993) 'Panic Diaries: (Re)Constructing a Partial Politics and Poetics of Disease' in J. Holstein and G. Miller (eds) *Reconsidering Social Constructionism: Debates in Social Problems Theory*, Aldine DeGruyter, New York.

Radley A. (ed.) (1993) *Worlds of Illness: Biographical and Cultural Perspectives on Health and Disease*, London/New York, Routledge.

Schou K.C. and Hewison J. (1999) *Experiencing Cancer: Quality of Life in Treatment*, Buckingham/Philadelphia, Open University Press.

Seale C. (1998) *Constructing Death: The Sociology of Dying and Bereavement*, Cambridge, Cambridge University Press.

Small N. and Rhodes P. (2000) *Too Ill to Talk? User Involvement and Palliative Care*, London/New York, Routledge.

Sontag S. (1991) *Illness as Metaphor – Aids and its Metaphors*, London, Penguin.

Stacey J. (1997*) Terratologies – A Cultural Study of Cancer*, London/New York, Routledge.

Werbner P. (1997) 'Introduction: The Dialectics of Cultural Hybridity' in P. Werbner and T. Modood (eds) *Debating Cultural Hybridity: Multicultural Identities and the politics of Anti-Racism*, London/New Jersey, Zed Books, 1–26.

Williams S.J. (2000) 'Chronic Illness as biographical disruption or biographical disruption as chronic illness? Reflections on a core concept', *Sociology of Health and Illness*, vol. 22, 1: 40–67

Winter H., Cheng K.K., Cummins C. *et al.* (1999) 'Cancer incidence in the South Asian population of England (1990-92)', *British Journal of Cancer*, 79 (3/4): 645–54.

Yates P. and Stetz K.M. (1999) 'Families' awareness of and response to dying', *Oncology Nursing Forum*, 26, 1: 113–20.

3

Identity and belief within black Pentecostalism: spiritual encounters with psychiatry

Gerard Leavey

Introduction

Over the past 30 years, studies in the UK consistently show higher rates of psychotic illness among African-Caribbeans, in turn prompting an expanding list of putative explanations for this overrepresentation which include genetic predisposition, the effects of migration, cannabis use, urbanisation, social disadvantage, racism and racial bias in the diagnostic practices of psychiatrists and the way life stresses are perceived and interpreted (King *et al.* 1994; Sharpley *et al.* 2001; Gilvarry *et al.* 1999). In addition, the presentation of mental illness may differ between cultures and ethnic groups and the use of diagnostic categories in Western psychiatry may overlook important cultural distinctions in the presentation of psychological distress (Littlewood and Lipsedge 1981; Fabrega 1989). Embedded within these cultural differences, religious identity and belief play a determining role in the type of relationship that black people have with psychiatric services. When religious patients and their families are pushed into contact with a secular psychiatry that tends to see religious belief as part of the patient's problem, either as cause or in presentation – a mutual suspicion strains the relationship.

In this chapter I am interested in the identity and beliefs of black people within the Pentecostal churches in the UK. It is argued that Pentecostalism's emphasis on family and community stability underpins the construction of a positive identity and may alleviate some of the insecurities and threats that percolate from migration upheaval, confronting the unknown and racism (Martin 2002). However, there are a number of contradictions within Pentecostalism, which provoke questions about the relationship between Pentecostal identity, belief and mental health. First, Pentecostalism is generally presented as a well-tested vehicle for the continuity of identity in a plethora of ethnic groups and cultures and is therefore acknowledged as a religion with the facility to absorb, adapt and manage diverse beliefs. Intrinsic to Pentecostalism is the transformation of the individual as they move from one identity to another, a rejection of the past, which may include family and friends.

Are Pentecostals more likely to develop mental health problems? There is a large body of research, mostly from the US, that suggests that church attendance, generally, is positively associated with greater emotional health explained by the promotion of resilience and the avoidance of negative exposures. Thus, the values of religious organisations are thought to promote healthy lifestyles (around sexuality, alcohol and drug use), the maintenance of social integration and mutual support, and the provision of reciprocal emotional and practical assistance (Maton 1987). Private worship may also promote sound mental health through meditation, connectedness to 'a divine order' and positive coping styles (Ellison and George 1994). It is not, however, all good news for the religious. Religion has been accused of suppressing self-esteem, crushing identity (e.g. ethnic minorities, women, homosexuals) and the manufacture of guilt-ridden, overly controlled neurotics (Freud 1930). In any case, an incisive review of the epidemiological evidence by Levin urges caution about the hitherto positive interpretations on religion and mental health. The issue of measurement of religion and spirituality is a long-standing block to interpretation (Levin 1994). Some evidence suggests that members of the Pentecostal churches in general are more likely to develop mental health problems than people from other faiths (Koenig *et al.* 1994). It has been posited that enthusiastic recruitment by Pentecostals among the marginalised, socially and psychologically distressed, in effect, creates a pooling of vulnerable people not found among more static, mainstream religious groups (Koenig 1994). For Pentecostalism in the UK (as elsewhere), migrant groups are a rich source of recruitment; and migrants, contingent on certain factors, are generally accepted as being more vulnerable to mental illness. However, there is little epidemiological evidence to support higher rates within black African migrants to the UK and it would seem that the incidence of mental disorder based on religion or strength of religious belief is unlikely to be available for calculation.

William James (1902) was one of the first to observe greater psychopathology among people with sudden conversion experience and, as I discuss, dramatic change, not confined to religion, which is usually taken as one facet of identity, forms a central element in the life of Pentecostalists. Nevertheless, it has been suggested that in transforming the identities and life trajectories of the excluded and oppressed, Pentecostalism provides a healing that is both social and spiritual, promising rewards expected by the individual both here and beyond. But here too at the bridge between this world and the anticipated next, Pentecostalism carries within it the possibilities of both healing and illness. There are aspects of Pentecostal identity and belief, which erase or at least, blur, the boundaries between natural and supernatural spheres and which may heighten conflict and anxieties about the origins of disease and suffering, in turn, generating a vulnerability to mental health problems.

In this chapter, I examine the literature on Pentecostalism and mental health, which combines sociological perspectives on religion, ethnicity and identity and anthropological and epidemiological research and theory on religion, health and healing. I include preliminary findings from recent epidemiological research and also from qualitative research that I am undertaking in London on the interface between religious organisations and psychiatric services. This work includes interviews with religious leaders from faith organisations, including Pentecostalist ministers, African and African-Caribbean. In addition I examine the work of a black assertive outreach team and the issues related to working with Pentecostalist patients and their families.

Religious identity and mental health

Religious-based beliefs held by people with mental health problems may influence help-seeking and compliance with treatment (Chadda et al. 2001; Cinnirella and Loewenthal 1999). Thus many patients who perceive their psychological problems as being spiritual or religious in origin will tend to seek religious support prior to, and often in place of, seeking help from orthodox psychiatric care (Narrow et al. 1993; Cole et al. 1995). From a psychiatric pathways study (Cole et al. 1995) and from interviews with carers prior to a family intervention study (Leavey et al. 2004), we found that religious organisations can play a mediating or obstructive role. Many of the black patients and their families, African and African-Caribbean, held strong connections with Pentecostal churches which influenced the patients and their families' help-seeking. It is alleged that some Pentecostalist groups, following the recruitment of people with mental health problems, encourage them to reject medical treatment in the pursuit of a new identity backed by commitment and faith (Diakonia 2003).

In an increasingly pluralist society, the desire and the ability of psychiatric services to respond to the needs of diverse communities is a contentious issue but cannot be ignored. In North London, 86 per cent of patients with first episode of psychosis had one or both parents born outside the UK (King et al. 1994). Mainstream Christian churches accounted for only 34 per cent of the religious faiths of patients in this sample and 44 per cent believed in witchcraft and also spirit possession. Indeed, 18 per cent of patients, and a similar proportion of their relatives, claimed to have personally experienced the effects of spirit possession. Many of these patients and their relatives attributed the occurrence of mental illness to 'spiritual' phenomena. A similar pattern of belief was observed in a community-based study of non-psychiatric individuals ($n = 428$) from the same area where two thirds of respondents aligned themselves with a religion or belief (MORI 1994). White people were considerably more likely to report having no faith than Black or Asian people (46 per cent compared with 11 per cent and 4 per cent respectively). Black and Asian residents were more likely to be actively religious than their white counterparts. More than a quarter of residents claimed to believe in supernatural forces and 23 per cent stated a belief in spirit possession, while 18 per cent believed in witchcraft. Of the Black group, 40 per cent claimed to believe in witchcraft and a similar proportion of Asians believed in spirit possession. Using a case-control method we explored the possibility that the excess incidence of psychosis among ethnic minority groups, particularly in African-Caribbeans, might be explained by the stronger presentation to services by this group with spiritual or religious beliefs (King *et al.* 2003). We found that ethnicity lost statistical significance as a predictor for psychotic illness after accounting for life events and spiritual beliefs. These findings raise the possibility that the explanation for higher rates of diagnosed psychotic illness among black people may be related to a greater experience of stress that leads to such disorders and because their particular expression of stress is misinterpreted as illness by a culturally ignorant psychiatric system. In inner-city areas with large minority ethnic populations and high rates of schizophrenia and other psychoses, strongly held religious identity and the attendant beliefs, likely to influence the presentation, help-seeking, treatment and outcomes of severe mental illness.

Continuity

It is commonly supposed that black Christian arrivals to Britain in the 1950s, and afterwards, were effectively and affectively turned away by a cold, white Christian climate to find refuge within churches that were more capable of articulating their needs and embracing their humanity. This is only partly true. African-Caribbean and other black migrants arrived in Britain armed with their own strong religious identity shaped by an African cultural inheritance, slavery and colonialism (Toulis 1997). In the slave community, the religious belief system of Obeah–Myal offered a system of 'explanation, prediction and control' that helped regulate social relations through the intervention of spirits (Horton 1967). Toulis suggests that in the context of slavery, the complex pantheon of spirits, deities and ancestors originating in West Africa was reduced to a general dichotomised belief of good and evil spirits. The Obeah practitioner used an armamentarium of incantations, charms, fetishes and poisons to dispense punishment, find wrongdoers or restore health (Williams 1933) while Myal provided a counterbalancing force. The black churches in Jamaica evolved with a more syncretistic character in both organisation and practice with teaching provided within smaller groups led by charismatic individuals chosen for their supernatural gifts and who exercised considerable power over group membership which was based on the ability of the applicant to demonstrate spirit possession, often induced by fasting and intense prayer, through the manifestation of visions and dreams. Revivalism, Toulis suggests was the result of the syncretism of Christianity and Myalism, characterised by highly dramatic and emotional displays of belief and worship such as dancing, falling prostrate, prophesying, trance and spirit possession; an emotionalism which became a permanent feature of Jamaican-African Christian cults (Curtain 1955). Toulis argues that although the sects and cults held little social prestige, they were able to meet the emotional and spiritual needs of the people. African-Christian sects not only offered explanations of suffering but also provided an otherwise un-empowered people with a system of practice through which they might seek to control the unpredictable and make reparations for perceived injustices (Toulis 1997).

In his examination of the West African experience, Hunt suggests that in addition to continuity, the Pentecostalist framework provides the West African migrants to Britain and elsewhere the basis 'to explore reflexively personal and social change'. As one of my respondents in this study puts it, a young lay pastor from Nigeria, 'My belief in God through Pentecostalism gives me the strength to put aside all concerns about racism and all the other things that can hold you back. With his love I can break free from all these things. My colour and my background are not important. I can be what I want to be through God'. This echoes Gifford's account of the success of Pentecostalism in West Africa as it nurtures a sense of self worth and an escape from helplessness (Gifford 1994). As Mol puts it with regard to sectarian religiosity, 'it is not just a means for better coping with existence but more fundamentally, a *relevant* way of coping with that existence' (Mol 1976:181).

Identity and mental illness

In establishing identity we map out boundaries, consciously and unconsciously, creating distinctions between those who belong and those who don't: 'them' and 'us'. It also involves classification – assigning and grouping according to a set of assumed and agreed sets of characteristics and behaviours often formed on a set of positive-negative dualisms. Central to any discussion of identity is that of the extent to which people are free to shape, own and control their identities as opposed to how identity is formed and manipulated by external forces at the social, political, economic and cultural level (Woodward 2000). Giddens, in discussing agency and structure, stresses that the autonomy of the self as an agent is about producing accounts of oneself (1991). Where then is the ability of the 'mad' to produce such accounts? Historically, these accounts have been invalidated.

We can assume that to some extent, aspects of personality (and thus identity) are genetically determined but leave the individual sufficient agency to shape the narrative. However, there are always significant exceptions to this plasticity. Madness, within most of Western culture at least, has been perceived both as loss and followed by loss; quarantine through banishment and exile, a commonplace sanitising response by the majority. The ability of the labelled mad to make rational choices and decisions is removed socially, both informally and in law. Agency is removed and arguably, also identity. We commonly speak of 'losing the mind', 'not the same person'; euphemistic legal language such as 'diminished responsibility' places the individual exterior to conventional punishment but repositions such people in a limbo state of literal and metaphorical incarceration. This repositioning of the individual's social identity brings with it enormous negative implications for his or her future. For Andrew Sims, the psychiatrist, continuity is a fundamental human need around which we base the healthy self. 'I am who I was last week, or thirty years ago; I am who I will be next week or in ten years' time. This truism, which we can claim without hesitation, is by no means certain for those suffering from schizophrenia or from organic states, from neuroses or depression or even from some healthy people in abnormal situations (*possession states*)' (Sims 1995).

Black and other ethnic minority groups, often migrants from former colonial states, have to contend with a rupture to continuity as they struggle to maintain core elements of past identity, provided 'at home' while attempting to fit on required but unfamiliar identities (or, familiar but rejected identities) in the new country (Fanon 1952). The ability of minority ethnic individuals and groups to resist or manage unwanted assigned identities depends on political and socio-economic factors. Nevertheless, Hall (1996) rightly argues that the production of cultural identity is an ongoing, fluid process within which a number of sociologists locate religion as a significant contributor in identity construction. Pentecostalism offers continuity and in doing so it helped resolve the difficulty of social and personal identity for African-Caribbeans and Africans in Britain. There are a number of significant and defining features of Pentecostalism, which enabled the new religion to brush aside racial, linguistic and cultural barriers and may be considered as possessing salutiferous effects for the individual and society. Seymour, an African-American, the founder of Pentecostalism, was committed to the ideal of inter-racial harmonisation within a segregated America. For Beckford (1998) the holiness teaching of speaking in tongues represented, literally as well as metaphorically, the possibility, at least, of an eradication of social division across all strata. At the social level, Pentecostalism is a church that provides sanctuary for the vulnerable exposed to racial exclusion. Within the UK, as elsewhere, it continues to provide an encompassing identity for marginalised black migrant groups and offers a solution to personal and group, past and present suffering. It is this transforming radicalism that has proved so successful for the Pentecostal movement in that it is careful to incorporate aspects of existing indigenous cultural identity while eschewing the less desirable. Thus for women in South America and elsewhere, oppressed by poverty, and unfaithful feckless husbands, the chance for a new identity and earthly salvation prior to the heavenly one, one might imagine to be an attractive proposition (Burdick 1993). Burdick suggests the primary reason for the rapid growth of Pentecostalism among Brazil's urban poor as tied to issues of community, an attempt to re-create some sense of order, identity and belonging. Similarly, d'Epinay (1969) sees the value of Pentecostalism to its adherents as an attempt to counteract the anomic forces of modernism and urbanisation, a crisis-adaptation model.

Encounters

Pentecostalism has sufficient ideological flexibility to eclectically accommodate local social conditions and culture. Indeed, some of the phenomenal growth of Pentecostalism has been attributed to it being a 'movement organisation' rather than the static, centralised, bureaucratic denominations (Gerlach and Hine 1970). The distinctive characteristics include 'a reticulate or polycephanous organisation linked together by a variety of personal, structural and ideological ties' (Gerloff 1992). It is therefore a migrant, highly portable mission that travels within existing social and kinship networks, flexible and unburdened by rigid hierarchies and bureaucracies; prepared to 'rough it'. Perhaps not surprisingly their developmental pathways and experiences reflect those of the migrant. Thus, many of the new urban Pentecostalist congregations are housed within makeshift buildings in the centre of poor urban communities. Van Dijk (2002) suggests that Pentecostal groups have become a prominent part of the migration process itself.[1]

Such is the rapid proliferation and diversity of Pentecostalism that it would be unwise to suggest the existence of a unified position on mental illness and certainly many of the older African-Caribbean churches distance themselves from the beliefs and practices of the newer, more vibrant African churches (usually Ghanaian or Nigerian). The range of opinions articulated by different Pentecostal pastors suggest no particular central ideology but rather a mixture of individual voices, reinforcing the sense of an organisation spreading through the individual, often idiosyncratic, will of energetic preachers. Nevertheless, there appears a nucleus of Pentecostalist ontological belief, influential on matters of illness, threaded through the mission of disparate churches. There is insufficient space here to give little more than a superficial outline of these relevant aspects but briefly they are:

1. an apocalyptic vision of the world; a fearful acceptance of the undeniable, ubiquitous presence of satanic forces in the universe that unceasingly employ all means to thwart God's message of salvation. Thus, the world is constantly in an agitated, expectant state; in the grip of total war largely played out behind the occult screen that separates our material world from the supernatural domain;

2. the existence and pre-eminence of a spirit world, hidden but active within all human behaviour and human events; thus biological explanations for illness and misfortune are generally inadequate in that a medical causal chain offers no place for spiritual intrusion along the pathway;
3. a religious worship that is individually and collectively profoundly experiential and beliefs that are not compartmentalised but 'lived' and constant.

Harvey Cox sees Pentecostal spirituality as a trifocal quest to recover a primal spirituality that had been abandoned or forgotten within mainstream Christianity. First, the individual, through deep personal piety, made manifest through dreams, visions and healing can rediscover this primal spirituality. Second, a recovery of primal hope within the millennial vision; that is, a certainty that a new age is imminent despite the confusion and distraction of the material universe (Cox 1996). The final part of this trinity of recovery was speaking in tongues, a return to pre-Babel *speech from the heart*. It is these aspects of Pentecostal belief, worship and identity, entwined with African and Caribbean culture generally, which are likely to be interpreted pathologically by Western atheistic psychiatry. I now illustrate some of these issues through the use of material gathered from the in-depth interviews.

Pastor S has been living and working in London for 23 years. His church, The Church of the Anointing Christ, part of the Elim Pentecostal ministries, is established above a vacant department store. Despite the relatively humble building environment, his office resembles that of a business executive, expensive telephony equipment, decked out with laptop and desktop computers, television screens and soft leather furnishings. The ability of Pentecostalism to manage the contradiction of unease with modernity while usefully availing itself of modernity's technology has been remarked upon by others (Wacker 1986). The impression given by the pastor is that he is as much in contact with the greater universe as he is with his flock in dilapidated Tottenham. He speaks with an accent that could be from Africa, England or North America. In fact, Pastor S came to London from Ghana and his congregation are mostly Ghanaians, although there are some English and 'Afro-Caribbean' but mostly Ghanaian because 'you build from a position of strength – it is easier to attract people from your own background'. He describes how the work of his church is not solely 'within church' but reaches out to people who need to hear the message of God. He also informed me that a great deal of the work of the church is attended to by small prayer groups of family and neighbours described as a process akin to cell division; in fact, the pastor refers to them as 'home cells'. Held in people's houses during weekdays, they are of help to people who have problems but are shy and unable to air them in public. For recent arrivals too, given the large migrant population associated with the Pentecostal movement, the small group provides acceptance and antidote to isolation providing a supportive, more intimate milieu, allowing people to share their burdens – a home. However, as with most organisations and groups, the social protection offered to the individual is often offset by a sacrifice of individual identity and maintenance of group loyalty policed by the group. The Pentecostal message is often one of liberation but the structures produce control. The smaller cell offers less opportunity for the doubter to drift, close bonding making it difficult to pull away from the church – the greater the intimacy, the greater the betrayal of leaving.

The pastor describes the way of worship within his church as

> Free style worship. Expressing worship to God in a more open, unreserved kind of way, and just flowing with the Holy Spirit because we believe in the Holy Spirit moving amongst the people ... they can express themselves more publicly in their worship to God.

Pastor S's language is full of militaristic imagery and metaphors. Words like 'arena', 'power', 'destruction', 'enemy', 'battle' and 'defeat' are used constantly. He describes how, following the expulsion from the garden of Eden, humans are obliged to live on earth in a parlous state – our souls need spiritual sustenance just as our bodies need food

> When the fish is out of water, it dies – it's cut off from its source. Man must also be with God, for when he is alienated or cut off from God, he dies.

Within the pastor's worldview, this is not just a loss of spirituality and the beginning of a spiritual death, but a material death also.

The Pentecostalist vision rejects a construction of illness as a random genetic (in biological terms), misfortune experience. With sufficient investigation behind the material appearance or manifestation, one can discern other covert forces in operation, underpinned or provoked by spiritual disturbance. The disturbance may have arisen by the individual's sinful actions or through the actions of others; thus the individual may be being punished for some past transgression within the family or suffering the consequences of a curse generated through the jealousy of others. People may inherit a curse in the same way that they may inherit an illness. The pastor in a search for a pattern of illness will ask 'why this person, why this illness?' It is important to stress that none of the Pentecostal ministers, similar to all other religious leaders interviewed, deny the reality of an illness and nor would they advise against the sick person contacting their doctor but emphasise the need for spiritual consultation when there is an underlying spiritual problem. This tends to be more strongly expressed by the Ghanaian pastor but articulated nevertheless by the others.

> Well medically speaking, there is some form of deficiency or something that has happened that caused their mental illness. From a doctor's point of view or an insurance point of view we would want to ask certain questions. When insurance has been taken out, they (the insurance company) ask whether a particular disease is found in the family, a condition is in the family because they believe that the likelihood of picking that up is strong because it can be traced in the family. So therefore, one can look at these sort of factors medically, but when we look at it spiritually the diagnosis comes back the same; when there's a frequent occurrence of a particular thing then you can begin to look at it almost as a spiritual activity.

For some of the ministers there is a difficulty in differentiating between mental illness and spiritual phenomena in that they are not seen as mutually exclusive entities. For Pastor S, mental illness may be a result of demon possession or may, as human weakness, leave open a portal, 'openings' as he describes them, for the entry of demons:

> A demon is this disembodied spirit. They want to be in a body and that is what Satan promised them. God has created the man and that man has a house, the flesh. So the desire of every demon is to go into a person. Now when a demon gets into a person – I mean there are many ways a demon can come in – a lot of the root causes, a lot of the problems is associated with mental illness or mental situation. From the spiritual perspective this is demons or spirits entered into bodies and the spirit can enter because the spirit is just air. There are different categories of demons and the type of things that they do, demons of lies, demons of hatred. People begin to manifest a particular way of a demon – maybe lies for example, spirit personality. Sometimes they are unaware of what is done until they come back to their senses – demons crave to come into bodies and I believe that when Satan promised them bodies or to be able to create doors for them to come into bodies then they went for it and so they looked for openings that they can come into a person. Now these openings are a lot, through generational and through ancestral and so that is why demons enter into a person and then take over when we say a person's possessed.

Birgit Meyer, from her ethnographic study on Ghanaian Christianity stresses the centrality of the devil in the Pentecostalist imagination and its omnipresence in public culture and space. Her description is often evocative of nation state propaganda in preparation for war or invasion, exhorting the population to hypervigilance or to suffer the catastrophic consequences (Meyer 2001). Thus, much more 'energy and passion' is put into the imagination of evil than into the imagination of good. Among other reasons, this emphasis on Satan and the boundary between Christianity and heathenism (traditional gods) gave Pentecostalism a big advantage over the other Christian mission churches in the recruitment and retention of souls. According to Meyer, while competing Christian churches in Ghana responded to the expansionist Pentecostalist threat by an Africanisation of the liturgy, Pentecostalism, ostensibly opposed to Africanisation, was in reality closer to African traditional worship. By relocating the old gods and spirits within the satanic camp and energetically fighting to remove them, they maintained a link with an African identity that 'softer' Christian groups attempted to cleanse from their own Eurocentric vision of Christianity. Pastor G confirms that the emergence of Pentecostalism within West Africa was not brought about through the rejection of 'old spirits and demons'; they still exist but have much less potency relative to the Christian God.

Pastor F is also from Ghana and has lived in London for 24 years. He has been a chaplain for the local psychiatric hospital. While less preoccupied by the workings of the devil than Pastor S he nevertheless detects the work of the devil in mental illness and places great emphasis of the confluence of spirit and body. He explains that while the spirit may not directly create injury, the spirit may be attacked, sometimes injuring the body. He relates the story of a female member of his congregation who dreamed one night of being stabbed. The following day, while recalling the dream to her friend, she became ill and was taken to hospital where she died. Pastor F believes that 'her spiritual side was attacked – whatever attacks the spirit effects the body'. The connection between these happenings is transparent. Likewise he is convinced that the difference between psychiatric and spiritual phenomena is thin and he would have little problem in seeing this:

> I have been chaplain for this hospital for 10 years and I've been meeting such problems. I didn't understand it because we, especially in our culture, when somebody's schizophrenic we think it is the devil. I have been explaining this to the nurses and that is why I used to say to them in hospital that you should recognise more the spirituality. There was an incident in one of the wards, there was a Rastafarian and they (the nurses) told me that every time I come to the ward he started calming down. So you see that there's something there.

The pastor explains that there exist three entities; the soul, the body and the spirit 'and the soul is between the body and the spirit'. When one's spiritual side is strong the soul will rise to the spirit but 'if you are more loose, then the soul will be dragged to the body side'. He goes on to explain that in

Africa if a person is seen to be possessed, a fetish priest is called and very often the victim will be chained up and denied food. In this understanding, in which the pastor appears to embrace certain aspects of traditional intervention, humans are in a constant tug of war, a zero-sum equation thus 'when the body is not receiving the food, the spirit is being filled – it's being made strong because when you fast, the body loses and the spirit gains'.

Pastor T migrated from Jamaica more than 40 years ago and has a small congregation on the outskirts of London. Most of his church members are from a Caribbean background and a smaller number from Africa. His beliefs about severe mental illness are more congruent with mainstream religious leaders in that he gives greater emphasis on the personal-social origins of disorder. While not excluding a spiritual component of illness, he provides a stress explanation. He is concerned that many young black people are misdiagnosed because of their behaviour, culturally acceptable among African-Caribbeans but misinterpreted and punished by psychiatrists:

> They might shout and they might speak in an aggressive manner and half the time, the things that they say, they don't really mean them but they only say it in the heat of the moment ... but because there's anger inside. We just don't think that it's quite right to brand them that way.

His thoughts about the treatment of young black people by the 'system' echo the concerns of the wider black community, which to some extent prompted the setting up of a multi-disciplinary team to manage the mental health problems of this group. Antenna, established in North London in 1999, is a mental health service based on the assertive outreach model, gaining recognition as an effective way to therapeutically engage people with severe and complex mental health problems. What is unique about this service, in the UK at least, is that it was established to serve the needs of young black people, mostly at early onset of psychotic illness, and provided by an interdisciplinary team of black mental health workers. What is also special about this team and the way they work is their attempt to engage a range of black community organisations and, particularly, church groups and their leaders. The reason for this is simple. It stems from a pragmatic recognition that the churches play an influential part in community life and the lives of almost one third of the clients of the service. To exclude religious participation and intervention might be to risk alienating patient, family and pastor. In some respects this therapeutic team attempt to provide solutions to mental health problems, which attempt an accommodation of certain aspects of social and religious identity and the beliefs that stem from the full spectrum of realities held by their patients. M is a qualified and experienced social worker in her 30s and has been working for Antenna for the past two years. An African-Caribbean woman, she was brought up as a Methodist but she attends a

Baptist church that sits within the Pentecostal and charismatic framework. She explains that the search for an authentic identity for Pentecostalists is 'walking the Christian walk', a demonstration of belief in everyday life in a manner that is truly consistent with the self and where one presents one face, 'being real'. The expression feels simultaneously both contemporary and old-fashioned.

> You know the miracles talked about within the bible are very much of the walking theme. Pentecostals apply the word of God to the present day. It's not like some story in the bye and bye. It's the same God that's worked miracles, turned water into wine, can do things today within your life and I've proved it for myself. This is not something that I'm just talking about. I've prayed and seen my prayers answered. I've done things and asked the Lord to show me signs and I've seen it happen you know so it's not something that is abstract – it's a part of me.

M also stresses the social closeness that she and her black colleagues have with the young black clients. They understand the difficulties of the neighbourhood but they also know the religious and spiritual issues, the significance that these hold, and how they are open to misinterpretation. From her work over the years with various mental health services in London she is concerned about the suppression of religious and spiritual beliefs held by the patients and carers; patients from a Pentecostalist background are anxious about being perceived as religious by psychiatry.

> People who had been through the system for a long time tended to keep quiet about it. It was such a shame because the church made a valid contribution to their lives but they kept it a secret because they thought they would be punished for it if they started to talk about their Christian walk, about their spiritual belief about feeling that they were possessed ... about the church actually.

> I was told when I working within the mental health system a lot of the times the clients will be talking about their spiritual walk and it will be seen as a form of madness and not a form of reality and you know, there was a lack of understanding so that was very heart rending for me ... the thing with the mental health system is that they never respect the patients' spirituality. Within ward rounds, the psychiatrist and the other staff are totally dismissive of the spiritual walk, which the client or the family is saying 'this is what has helped us, this is what's carried us through' ...

Walking the spiritual walk is an integral element of the Pentecostalists existence (or considered as the existence itself) but there are boundaries of identity and behaviour that, when breached, bring the individual into personal danger. A key theme found within most religious leaders' conceptualisation of mental illness was that of an individual moving beyond accepted religious devotion to the detriment of family and other relationships; indeed, an attachment to religious ritual that betrays a spiritual and also psychological malaise. Thus for the person to step out of the parameters of his or her recognised identity through the neglect of self, duty and family, even if it is motivated by religious zeal, is perceived as indicating disintegration, a descent into malfunction. However, while most Christian and other religious leaders maintain a wary scepticism about individual claims to a special relationship and communication with God, detecting instead some degree of mental illness, the Pentecostalist ministers appear more ambivalent. In order to understand the uncertainty of the Pentecostalist ministers to definitively discriminate between spiritual and psychiatric phenomena, we need first to understand the fundamental characteristics of Pentecostal beliefs and worship. A number of factors attached to the quest for primal spirituality described by Cox are salient. First, some of the ambivalence emanates from a reluctance to discount the proximity and accessibility of the divine, and its supernatural corollary, the satanic, in the fabric of everyday life. For the Pentecostal believer, if supernatural activity is omnipresent in the everyday then 'unusual' events may not be considered 'accidental', creating a heightened vigilance for signs of supernatural activity of good or evil. Faith healings and exorcisms are regular features within Pastor S's church, indeed in many African Pentecostal churches, but less so in the African-Caribbean churches. Importantly, while mainstream religions have tended to shed emotional mysticism, within Pentecostalist congregations, an individual's identity and prominence is highly predicated upon an active ostentatious spirituality: ecstatic (literally meaning 'out of place') as opposed to static. Where to a large extent, mainstream religions expect quiet, private and internal devotion, Pentecostal worship is often both emotional and public. This very aspect of African-Caribbean cultural behaviour that Pastor F felt brought negative consequences and some commentators suggest, leads to higher rates of involuntary psychiatric admission.

Central to Pentecostalism is the presence of the Holy Spirit manifested through the gifts of healing, speaking in tongues (glossolalia) and prophecy, all located in the human body (Droogers 1999). These gifts, or charismata, which can be obtained by the faithful through conversion and baptism in the spirit, confer on the individual a special position within the congregation, a contribution to their identity and belonging. The conversion experience, or breakthrough, is perceived and felt and often described as 'rebirth'. In this dramatic event, the converted shift to a truly radically new position, a rupture with their previous identity and beliefs (Hexham and Poewe 1997). The individual obtaining the power of the Holy Spirit is empowered to solve all manner of existential problems and this remains 'a healing resource in the ongoing struggle for life' (Droogers 1999). Furthermore, within the duality of the Pentecostalist *weltanshaaung* the convert has moved from the domain of the satanic to that of God and is required to be active in the struggle for hegemony on earth. Thus, spiritual safety demands constant vigilance and proselytisation; the insidious work of Satan must be revealed and the world warned. As Droogers points out, the conversion experience demands that a person rejects those cultural customs considered by Pentecostalism as sinful and demonic. Kinship ties are often broken and new loyalties formed. Again, we encounter one of the many paradoxes contained within Pentecostalism; offering continuity through the wrench of migration but nevertheless ready to insist on the amputation of previous identity. Poloma's insider account of the benefits of Pentecostalism goes further. Blending Victor Turner's 'dramaturgical paradigm' and aspects of symbolic interactionism, Poloma observes in Pentecostal worship a powerful impact on self-formation, identity and character. Her interviewees describe dramatic, ecstatic transformation from a life of defeat and hopeless low self-esteem to one that shines with courage and hope (Poloma 1997:8).

When working with families of Pentecostal patients, the Antenna team strive to find a mediating path between the secular modus operandi of modern psychiatry and the spiritual needs and demands of the patient, family and their pastors who often take a close supervisory position in the patient's care. It is quite usual for family pastors to sit in on case conferences, either at the family's request or, where difficult negotiation is expected, through invitation by the care team. The staff must negotiate and manage the extent to which religious healing such as prayer and fasting can intrude into the lives of their clients. M's position is that people can take their

> Christian walk out of context, take it to extremes to the detriment of their mental health ... respecting their thing so much that they're killing themselves.

She describes situations she encountered in previous social work posts where families acting on their beliefs have chained up a mentally ill relative in a prayer house but she is clear that this is not something that has been approved of in the bible.

> His family couldn't get treatment for him ... because his presentation was very violent, very psychotic, hearing voices, auditory and visual hallucinations. Their perspective (his family, church, etc) was that this man was possessed ... so the only way they could contain him and his violent behaviour ... they chained him up in a prayer house and they were praying over him thinking that was the only way.

N, the manager of Antenna, is not a Pentecostalist. She believes that young black people are over-represented in the psychiatric system, partly the result of discrimination in society but also because of misdiagnosis; an inability of psychiatry to cope with culturally determined behaviour, religious and otherwise. N gives a strong positive recognition of the work that the churches undertake within the black community such as their entrepreneurial drive in setting up luncheon clubs, after-school programmes, outreach projects with marginalised members of the community and pastoral counselling. Nevertheless, she must grapple with the difficulties created by the collision of religious beliefs and the medical needs of patients.

> I think the difference is they can hide their symptoms behind a religious ideology; so for instance if they have a particular delusion it is often hidden, it is often explained in a way related with their religious belief. So I think in that sense it makes them quite different and very much harder to work with. Sometimes you have a preacher present at the meeting who counters everything you say and that can be very difficult to manage in that situation.

Sometimes the ministers challenge the beliefs of staff, attempt conversion or try to persuade them to pray as part of the therapy.

> If you go in there and you have dreadlocks it will seem that you can't have the same belief system as them – so sometimes you have all these things being fought out and it is not always helpful. I think for the young person, because they are in a state of confusion, being pulled very much by the parents and the minister into one way of looking at their illness and sometimes it is just not helpful.

According to N, some of the pastors are able to tell the difference between mental illness and demon possession (although not discarding the concept of possession). They can discern this by how the person presents family background – if a person had been *hexed* or *obeahed* ...

> The way the preacher describes it, if you are in the light of a holy place and you are possessed by demons then that would manifest differently than if you just have an illness. I am not sure how that is presented but I think it's something to do with observation of fear, observation of how that person chants, they won't pick up the bible, they don't want you to quote, they scorn the holy water, lots of other things they'll pick up which says this is more than somebody being with a mental illness.

M has an assessment of the origins and characterisation of what is a malevolent supernatural power which I would suggest is significant within the historical and current context of the African-Caribbean community. She stresses the avoidance of

> anything restrictive, or anything that is not free. The Lord Jesus Christ said 'I came to make you free', so anything that is controlled is witchcraft, that's what we learn as Pentecostal Christians ... if somebody is saying to you, you have to do this, you have to wear this colour, then it's not from God.

A leitmotif throughout the Pentecostalist literature, and which contains a significant emotional resonance for African-Caribbeans, is that of enslavement by Satan. It is a multi-symbolic language that both explains past and present oppression and offers a course for liberation and salvation for all.

Healing

> If I did feel someone was possessed I wouldn't be afraid to say it. You know that's how strong I believe in my faith. But in all my years that I've been a practitioner I cannot say that I have seen somebody that I feel has been possessed. However I do not believe as a Christian that sickness is not from the Lord because God gives us all good things – he says, I will give you the desires of your heart to make your joy complete in me and also he gives us good things so I believe that if you are afflicted with any illness than it is not from the Lord, it must be from the devil, yeah, that's any sickness. (M)

Ness (1980) suggests that the therapeutic effects of glossolalia and possession behaviour was due to three interacting factors: first, the attainment of social status and enhancement of self-esteem within the church community as 'God's spokesman'; second, the acting out of aggressive behaviour which is negatively sanctioned outside the church; and third, the relief of emotional tension through verbal expressions that do not reveal the personal source of those emotions to others in the congregation. Ness felt that participation in fundamentalist religious activities may have a beneficial effect on 'demoralised individuals', depressed, anxious individuals with poor self-esteem. The anthropologist Thomas Csordas concludes that the most common feature of healing forms is religious in nature (Csordas 1998) and it is not difficult to detect universal commonalities of process and function between Pentecostalist and other indigenous healing rituals (Dorta 1976; Gill 1977; Jilek 1982; Singer and Garcia 1989; Spickard 1991). Moreover, as the stigma of mental illness remains a potent negative feature of the lives of people with such conditions (Link *et al.* 1989; Angermeyer *et al.* 1987; Markowitz 1998), there are a number of ways in which the attribution to mental disorder of a religious causation may be of 'help' to the individual and his or her family. As in the case of a religious or spiritual explanation, the locus of control is external to the individual and thus removes responsibility or blame from that individual. It is possible that a religious explanation, free of a biological genetic connection, is preferable to a psychiatric diagnosis and thus less stigmatising; the focus is fixed on the individual not on the wider family. However, as has been noted, in Pentecostalism the individual's problem is often family owned, seen as the result of transgression by other family members in this or past generations. Nevertheless, a faith solution to a spiritually derived 'problem' such as possession may represent the possibility of a dramatic fix and an elevation in status. Where there is some acceptance of psychiatric diagnosis by families there often remains, as we have seen, a great reluctance to relinquish an intervention of healing through faith and the close involvement of the local church. In doing so, this can create delays to psychiatric treatment.

Conclusion

Religion can provide a bridge between individualist and collectivist identities and appears to give the individual a sense of direction, meaning and unity (Beit-Hallahmi 1989; Allport 1950). I would stress, therefore, that the purpose of this chapter has not been to pathologise Pentecostal beliefs and worship. As I have attempted to demonstrate, there is much in Pentecostalism that provides black people in the UK, as elsewhere, with a profound sense of renewed and revised identity and with this, a self-esteem that is able to emerge from a complex narrative that incorporates historical and present themes of suffering and redemption. At a time when Christianity appears to be in decline, the symbolism within Pentecostalism manages to tap into the concerns and fears of Africans and African-Caribbeans in the UK and perhaps provides solutions and healing that are dissonant with medicine and psychiatry which find little place for spirituality and religious faith (King and Dein 1998; Culliford 2002). As Atwood Gaines points out, there is a tendency within science and medicine to invalidate alternative worldviews by referring to them as 'beliefs'. Western beliefs about medicine are classified simultaneously as knowledge (Gaines 1998). It is unfortunate but perhaps inevitable that attempting to maintain a Pentecostalist identity through the expression of faith can bring the religious individual into conflict with non-religious psychiatric health professionals.

Historically, there has been a deep strain of reliance on divine healing and vociferous anti-medicine within Pentecostalism (Synan 2000). Additionally, the glorification of a religious experience that blurs into the diagnostic symptoms of psychotic illness is a dramatic and emotional type of religious behaviour that has provoked an embarrassed distancing from mainstream Christianity and is viewed in psychiatry as reasonable evidence of psychopathology. Schizophrenia, arguably the most destructive of the mental disorders, is presented in the Western medical paradigm as the fragmentation of the individual, 'a disconnection between thoughts, actions and feelings'. Pentecostalism sees unity and integration of human and spiritual identity, a convergence of body, mind and spirit through prophecy, dreams, visions and healing (Droogers 1994) – the very bricks and mortar of psychotic diagnosis. Pentecostal religious belief and experience represents for Droogers a critique of 'Western culture' or perhaps more accurately, modernity and Western Cartesian scientism. Thus, modernity's willingness to accept a plurality of truths and realities, an identity created through lifestyle choices is strongly opposed by the Pentecostal commitment to a single, unifying truthful identity achieved through the religious experience. Relativism in this worldview is simply wrong and reckless. Moreover, for Pentecostals, the Western existence is a compartmentalisation of religious, social and individual experience whereby the body, made separate from the mind and objectified by medical science, is independent from spiritual influence; the sacred is allocated a discrete time frame (Sunday) and social space (church) but lacks expression elsewhere; worship itself is mediated through the preacher – the laity denied access to the 'religious means of production', as Drooger puts it; dreams and visions can only be given sanctioned time and expression within psychotherapy. Put simply, Pentecostalism offers the individual the opportunity to transcend boundaries and restrictions, bringing the illuminating sacred into the drab corners of the everyday but in doing so runs the risk of having the person being labelled mad. The need for dialogue between psychiatric services and faith communities is crucial.

Notes

1. Van Dijk describes a prayer camp in Ghana led by a prophetess and Deacon of the church, Grace Mensah Adu. The camp attracts many thousands of people every year, in search of resolution to a wide range of illnesses, problems and misfortune. Many others come to the camp for help in overcoming the obstacles to migration to Europe and the west. Grace Mensah will conduct prayer sessions 'over passports, visas and air-tickets' and urges those who come for travel 'problems' to engage in dry fasting (no food or water). The purpose of which is to build the supplicant's spiritual powers in preparation for spirit visitation and eventual 'breakthrough'. Religion becomes the travel guide for both the earthly and the spiritual journey.

References

Allport G.W. (1950) *The individual and his religion*, New York, Macmillan.

Angermeyer M., Link B., Majcher-Angermeyer A. (1989) 'Stigma perceived by patients attending modern treatment centers: some unanticipated effects of community psychiatric reforms', *Journal of Nervous Mental Disorders*, 175: 4–11.

Beckford R. (1998) *Jesus is Dread: Black Theology and Black Culture*, London, Darton, Longmann and Todd, 9–10.

Beit-Hallahmi B. (1989) *Prolegomena to the psychological study of religion*, Lewisburg, PA, Bucknell University Press.

Burdick J. (1993) *Looking for God in Brazil; the progressive Catholic Church in Urban Brazil's Religious Arena*, Berkeley, CA: University of California Press.

Calley M. (1965) *God's People: West Indian Pentecostal Sects in England*, London, Oxford University Press.

Chadda R.K., Agarwal V., Singh M.C. and Raheja D. (2001) 'Help seeking behaviour of psychiatric patients before seeking care at a mental hospital', *International Journal of Social Psychiatry*, 47 (4), 71–8.

Cinnirella M. and Loewenthal K.M. (1999) 'Religious and ethnic group influences on beliefs about mental illness', *British Journal of Psychology*, 72, 505–54.

Cole E., Leavey G., King M. *et al.* (1995) 'Pathways to care for patients with a first episode of psychosis; a comparison of ethnic groups', *British Journal of Psychiatry*, 167, 6, 770–6.

Comas-Diaz (1981) 'Puerto Rican espiritismo and psychotherapy', *American Journal of Orthopsychiatry*, 51, 636–45.

Corten A. and Marshall-Fratani, R (eds) (1999) *Pentecostalism and Trans-nationalism*, London, Hurst.

Cox H. (1996) *Fire From Heaven*, London, Cassell.

Csordas T. and Lewton E. (1998) 'Practice, performance and Experience in Ritual Healing', *Transcultural Psychiatry*, vol 35(4): 435–512.

Culliford L. (2002) 'Spiritual care and psychiatric treatment: an introduction', *Advances in Psychiatric Treatment*, 8, 249–58.

D'epinay C.L. (1969) *Haven of the Masses; a study of the Pentecostal movement in Chile*, London, Lutterworth Press.

Diakonia (2003) Council of Churches – personal communication.

Droogers A. (1994) *The Normalisation of Religious Experience. in Charismatic Christianity as Global Culture*, Karla Poewe (ed.), University of South Carolina Press.

Ellison C.G. and George L.K. (1994) 'Religious involvement, social ties and social support in a southeastern community', *Journal for the Scientific Study of Religion*, 33, 46.

Fanon F. (1967) *Black Skin White Masks*, London, MacGibbon and Kee.

Fabrega H. (1989) 'Cultural relevatism and psychiatric illness', *Journal of Nervous and Mental Diseases*, 177: 415–25.

Freud S. (1930) *Civilisation and its Discontents,* London, Hogarth Press.

Furley O.W. (1965) 'Protestant missionaries in the West Indies: Pioneers of a Non-racial society', *Race*, vol 6, 3, 232–42.

Gaines A.D. (1998) 'Religion and Culture in Psychiatry: Christian and Secular Psychiatric Theory and Practice in the United States' in H.G. Koenig (ed.) *A Handbook of Religion and Mental Health*, Academic Press, California.

Geertz C. (1973) *The interpretation of cultures*, New York, Basic Books Inc.

Gerlach L.P. and Hine V.H. (1968) 'Five factors crucial to the growth and spread of a modern religious movement', *Journal for the Scientific Study of Religion*, 7: 23–40.

Gerloff R. (1992) *A Plea for British Black Theologies*, Frankfurt, Peter Lang, 23–48.

Giddens A. (1991) *Modernity and Self-Identity*, Cambridge, Polity Press.

Gill S. (1977) 'Prayer as Person: the performance force in Navajo prayer acts', *History of Religions*, 17, 143–57.

Gilvarry C.M., Walsh E., Samele C. *et al.* (1999) 'Life events, ethnicity and perceptions of discrimination in patients with severe mental illness', *Social Psychiatry and Psychiatric Epidemiology*, 34: 600–08.

Goater N., King M., Cole E. *et al.* (1999) 'Ethnicity and outcome of psychosis', *British Journal of Psychiatry*, 175, 34–42.

Hall S. (1996) 'Who needs identity' in S. Hall and P. du Gay (eds) *Modernity and Its futures*, Oxford, Polity Press.

Harrison G., Owens D., Holton A. *et al.* (1988) 'A prospective study of severe mental disorder in Afro-Caribbean patients', *Psychological Medicine*, 18, 643–57.

Hill C. (1971) 'From Church to Sect: West Indian Sect Development in Britain', *Journal for the Scientific Study of Religion*, vol 10.

Horton R. (1967) 'African Traditional Thought and Western Science' in B.R. Wilson (ed.) *Rationality*, Blackwell, Oxford.

Hunt S. (2002) 'Neither here nor there: The Construction of Identities and Boundary Maintenance of West African Pentecostals', *Sociology*, vol 36, (1) 147–69.

James W. (1902) *The Varieties of Human Experience: A Study in Human Nature*, New York, Random House.

Jilek W.G. (1983) *Indian healing: Shamanic ceremonialism in the Pacific Northwest today*, Blaine, Hancock House Publishers.

King M., Coker E., Leavey G. *et al.* (1994) 'Incidence of psychotic illness in London: comparison of ethnic groups', *British Medical Journal*, 309, 1115–19.

King M., Leavey G., Mann V. *et al.* (2003) 'Culture, ethnicity and psychosis: a population based, case-control study' (submitted).

King M. and Dein S. (1998) 'The Spiritual variable in psychiatric research', *Psychological Medicine*, 28, 1259–62.

Koenig H.G., George L.K., Meador K.G. *et al.* (1994) 'Religious Affiliation and Psychiatric Disorder among Baby Boomers', *Hospital and Community Psychiatry*, 45, 6, 586–96.

Levin J.S. and Vanderpool H.Y. (1987) 'Is frequent religious attendance really conducive to better health? Toward an epidemiology of religion', *Social Science and Medicine*, 7, 689–700.

Leavey G., Gulamhussein S., Papadopoulos C. *et al.* (2004) 'A Randomised Controlled Intervention for families of patients with a first onset of psychosis', in press.

Levin J.S. (1994) 'Religion and health: Is there an association, is it valid and is it causal?', *Social Science and Medicine*, 38, 1475–82.

Link B., Cullen F., Struening E. *et al.* (1989) 'A modified labeling theory approach in the area of the mental disorders; an empirical assessment', *American Sociological Review*, 54: 400–23.

Littlewood R., Lipsedge M. (1988) 'Psychiatric illness among British Afro-Caribbeans', *British Medical Journal*; 296: 950–1.

Markowitz F. (1998) 'The effects of stigma on the psychological well-being and life-satisfaction of persons with mental illness', *Journal of Health and Social Behaviour*, 39: 335–47.

Martin D. (2002) *Pentecostalism: The world their parish*, Oxford, Blackwell.

Maton K.I. (1987) 'Patterns and psychological correlates of material support within a religious setting: the bi-directional support hypothesis', *American Journal of Community Psychology*, 15, 185.

Meyer B. (2001) ' "You devil, go away from me!" Pentecostalist African Christianity and the Powers of Good and Evil' in P. Clough and J.P. Mitchell (eds) *Powers of Good and Evil; social transformation and popular belief*, London, Berghahn Books.

Mol H. (1976) *Identity and the Sacred: a sketch for a new social-scientific theory of religion*, Oxford, Blackwell.

MORI (1994) 'Haringey and Enfield Life Experiences; a survey of residents', research study conducted with St Ann's and Royal Free Hospitals First Onset Psychosis Research Team.

Narrow W.E., Reiger D.A., Rae D.S. *et al.* (1993) 'Use of services by persons with a mental and addictive disorders: findings from the National Institute of Mental Health Epidemiologic Catchment Area Program', *Archives of General Psychiatry*, 50, 85–94.

Ness (1980) 'The impact of indigenous healing activity: an empirical study of two fundamentalist churches', *Social Science and Medicine*, 14b,167–80.

Poewe K. (1989) 'On the Metonymic Structure of Religious Experiences: the example of charismatic Christianity', *Cultural Dynamic*, Vol 11, No. 4, 361–80.

Sharpley M., Hutchinson G., McKenzie K. and Murray R. (2001) *British Journal of Psychiatry*, 178 (suppl) s60–s68.

Sims A. (1995) *Symptoms in the Mind, an introduction to descriptive psychopathology*, London, Saunders.

Singer M. and Garcia R. (1989) 'Becoming a Puerto Rican espiritista: Life history of a female healer' in C.S. McClain (ed.), *Women as healers: In cross-cultural perspectives*, New Brunswick.

Spickard J. (1991) 'Experiencing religious rituals: A Schutzian analysis of Navajo ceremonies', *Sociological Analysis*, 52, 191–204.

Synan V. (2000) 'A Healer in the House? A historical perspective on healing in the Pentecostal/charismatic tradition', *Asian Journal of Pentecostal Studies*, 3.2.189–201.

Toulis N.R. (1997) *Believing Identity; Pentecostalism and the Mediation of Jamaican Ethnicity and Gender in England*, Oxford, Berg.

van Dijk R. (2002) 'The Soul is the Stranger: Ghanaian Pentecostalism and the diasporic contestation of "flow" and "individuality"', *Culture and Religion*, vol 3, 1, 49–65.

Wacker G. (1986) 'The Pentecostal Tradition' in R.L. and D.W. Amundsen (eds) *Caring and Curing: Health and Medicine in the Western Religious Traditions. Numbers*, New York, Macmillan.

Williams J.J (1993) *Voodoos and Obeahs*, New York, Dial Press.

Woodward K. (2000) *Questioning identity: Gender, Class, Nation*. London, Routledge.

Wuthnow R. (1993) *Christianity in the Twenty-first Century: Reflections on the challenge Ahead*. Oxford, Oxford University Press.

4

Identity and Alzheimer's disease

Jane Garner

'Can I have become a different person whilst remaining myself.'
Simone de Beauvoir

'I am' – the briefest but most powerful phrase in the language; whether spoken by self or by others, it is comforting and reassuring, also terrifying and unnerving. 'I am' begins the ten commandments (Exodus 20: 2) filling Moses with awe. The 'I am' of personhood is self and identity. At the heart of 'I am' is that non-trivial existential knowledge neither validated by external factors nor by others, that autonoesis about which we cannot be mistaken, have no ambiguity and which we assume is unique to humans. At the centre of humanhood is this knowledge of our own existence which requires neither explanation nor objective verification.

The word 'identity' comes from the Latin *identitas* meaning 'sameness'. The ultimate source being *idem*, 'same'; from *id*, 'it', 'that one'. The English descendant of this word is 'individuality' with the notion of something being itself rather than something else, always being the same. This identity sameness may be qualitative 'Bill and Ben have the same haircut' or quantitative/numerical 'Venice and Venezia are the same city'. Sameness can consist of having the same properties or being identifiable as the same thing even though many of its properties have changed. Many things persist through change in the natural and human world: the sapling becomes the tree; the child becomes the man. Judgements of identity involve assumptions about the nature of that to be identified. If my axe has a new head, is it then the same axe? If it subsequently needs a new shaft, will it then be the same axe? How much continuity is required for identity? Identities change over time. Am I the same 'I am' of 20, 30, 40 years ago? Am I the same 'I am' if I put on weight, dye my hair, have a limb amputated, drink alcohol or have a sex change operation? There is a sense of an unchanging core.

Alzheimer's disease with its progressive inevitable deterioration in memory, language and skills causes us to consider more the meaning of personhood and identity. Memory of who I am, even who I was, seems an important aspect of identity. Psychological continuity may be achieved through memory. How much memory is required to maintain identity and personhood? People change qualitatively with dementia; what degree of psychological continuity is sufficient to maintain quantitative identity? Memories are complex and usually unauthenticated. False memories are not held only by those who are psychologically disturbed, they are a feature of being human. Episodic memory may seem to be related to identity but cannot found the sense of self. Personhood presupposes a sense of self, an active identification with 'I am' that is immune from change. Is this sense of self so secure that it is resistant to the ravages of dementia? How many intact neurones are needed for 'I am'? Does identity shrink with the deterioration which comes with the disease? If identity shrinks, does it shrink to '*id*' – that primal, primitive, primary process, genderless, 'it'?

This chapter looks at the concept of identity as it relates to Alzheimer's disease, the most frequently occurring dementing illness, and considers the patient, their family, the staff employed and the societies in which the patients live.

Some philosophical considerations

John Locke (1632–1704) trained as a physician but subsequently gave more attention to politics and to philosophy than to medicine. He was the first of the British empiricists who took the view, denying innate knowledge, that all knowledge is derived from experience. It is the conscious self that is the person: without this thinking consciousness, there is no person (Locke 1690). He distinguishes between man, the human body and person, the conscious self. A person is someone who is conscious of their own existence; in this consists personal identity, 'without consciousness there is no person' (Lock 1690: 218). Links joining a person's former and current state maintains identity. The Lockean view raises many ethical questions about the unconscious patient and also about the one with severe dementia who may have no sense of continuity with their past self and so have lost Lockean personhood.

David Hume (1711–1776) initially studied law before turning his thinking to epistemology, ethics and philosophy. He considered that we need memory for notions of causation and effect which constitute the self, the person. By treating successive perceptions as though they were the same we create the fiction of personal identity over time. 'The identity which we ascribe to the mind of man is only a fictitious one' (Hume 1739:308); memory is the source of this personal identity. Derek Parfit is an Oxford philosopher, the thrust of whose work is towards a less self-centred outlook. He describes an individual as 'a descendant self' (Parfit 1971:21) who can think of any earlier incarnation as 'an ancestral self'. These states of self are transitive. For Parfit, having past and future selves, does not imply identity through time. There is no underlying 'I' person who is these successive selves.

In the Locke, Hume and Parfit tradition, a man could be a different person at different times. To be a person is to have psychological states; a reductive view that a person is no more than connected mental states. However, we continue to see the person who has severe dementia as continuing to exist and to behave in ways that are personal to them. Hughes (2001), in an elegant and compassionate paper, drawing also on his clinical work as an old-age psychiatrist, enlarges the view of personhood. A person is a 'situated-embodied-agent'. It is not possible to characterise psychological phenomena independent of the context in which they are embedded. We are 'situated' in a familial, cultural and historical context with lives as narrative and shape which contribute to our identity. 'Embodiment' adds to the narrative through bodily perceptions and experiences giving a psychobiographical shape and unity. Human beings are active 'agents' with a point of view and a purpose. In the Lockean view, the man with dementia is the same man but a different person to the one he was before the dementia, or not even a person at all. Hughes 'situated-embodied agent' description (Hughes 2001: 90) makes a presumption in favour of the person; also that the person is situated in a physical, emotional, conative and cognitive history; the person is embedded in a familial, social, professional context; and that the person is an agent and these agentive capabilities should be supported even when reduced by a dementing illness. The view that the person may survive into severe dementia put forward from a philosophical perspective by Hughes is echoed by psychodynamic psychotherapists (Garner 2004) who recognise that even into the late stages of the disease the ability to make a relationship is retained so that a therapeutic attachment may develop quickly.

The notion of concrete identity may be constraining for philosophers. Clinical intuition suggests that understanding the concrete rather than the philosophical/metaphysical identity of a person, their social context, history, personal commitments and values is essential to addressing real human and personal concerns which are brought to the consulting room. Personhood is held within life history and experience, in relationships and engagement with others. In this the person with dementia is no less a person than his neighbour or himself when well. The link between memory and personhood is weakened if identity at any given moment is not based on unchanging identity over time. Enduring 'I am' over time is not necessary for instantaneous 'I am' at a particular time. There is a temporal, longitudinal identity which may be explored in reminiscence work and moment-to-moment immediate identity which in a current social context may be investigated in intimate conversation or by empathic observation, e.g. dementia care mapping.

Society, identity, old age and dementia

Contemporary western society tends to conflate ideas of identity and of image. We are who we want to be or can afford to be. Cultural icons are young, fit, beautiful, 'fashionable'. We are self-absorbed but in an external self image of looks, clothes and inevitably youth. Goffman (1959) describes impression management – presenting identity as a series of masks depending on the audience. We become entranced by celebrity where the masks, expensive financially and personally, are of material wealth, special labels, re-fashioned bodies and 'the life fantastic'. In the post-modern aestheticism of everyday life, people make their lives into art assignments matching household goods and personal appearance. Life is seen as a cultural project. There is an increase in individualisation with individuals having less of a sense of belonging and embeddedness in local communities, families and social class. Identities tend to be based on lifestyle rather than class or nation and individuals rework their identities or image over time. Individualism is a key feature of Western culture. It is encouraged in a capitalist society with emphasis on the rights and freedoms of the individual in the hope that autonomous, enterprising individuals will create an eco-nomic free market. In a society which values youth, physical prowess and beauty, autonomy, independence, enterprise and productivity, it will be difficult to be old especially if one is old and ill. It can be seen as liberated to disrespect those groups and institutions previously regarded as having authority. Older people are caught up in this tide of apparent freedom but real chaos and ageism. There is a temporality to life; we progress through time to death. It is a conceptual strain to think of immortality – in those stories and legends where the protagonist cannot die (e.g. *The Flying Dutchman*, Wagner 1843) he is inevitably tormented and desperate for release. Life has a shape, a beginning, a middle and an end. Despite our knowledge of and to some extent comfort in this temporality and shape we nevertheless fear and hate old age. 'Every man desires to live long; but no man would be old', wrote Jonathan Swift (1667– 1745). Negative images of old age abound in literature and the arts. In Shakespeare's '*As you like it*' (II: vii), the last of the seven ages of man 'Sans teeth, sans eyes, sans taste, sans everything' seems grim indeed. To Dorian Gray (Wilde 1891), the idea of getting old was so terrifying he split off his ageing self and projected it into the loathed portrait kept out of view. Cosmetic surgeons now do the same for their customers – injecting, removing, implanting, to eradicate the signs of natural ageing.

Qualities or features admired in a young man are derided in the old. Designer stubble in the young is merely scruffy and unshaven in the old; low-crutched trousers in the young are fashion, in the old are simply ill fitting; what is considered virility at 25, becomes lechery at 65 (Berezin 1972). In the shape of life there may be modes of dress and behaviour more appropriate to one time than another but rarely do we congratulate people for ageing well, rather we applaud them for seeming younger than their years (Garner 2002) if they can 'carry it off', a confidence trick on others and themselves. Old people too, as part of society, enacting and internalising the role or identity they have been given, have conscious and unconscious negative images of themselves and their peers. Evans (1998) draws on the concept of malignant mirroring (Zinkin 1983) to explain the poor services expected by and provided to older people, it reflects a psychopathology of diminishment and imperfection.

It is not only individuals but also major politico-cultural forces which express negative opinions about older people who are considered to 'take' from the welfare system rather than to have made lifelong contributions, they are a 'burden' on the (inevitably younger) taxpayer. The Health Advisory service, one function of which is to advocate for patients, entitled one of its reports 'The Rising Tide' engendering images of the drowning of society by needy, engulfing old people. We place a lower value on the lives of older people and utilitarian calculations may influence our ethical stance towards them. Recently a London hospital in the midst of a bed crisis closed the Accident and Emergency Department to those over 70 who clearly presented problems too costly and too bothersome for the hard-pressed NHS. The post-modern promotion of self-reliance, competitiveness and the free market leaves little room for the chronic and multiple handicaps which accumulate for some in old age. Bell (1996) makes the point that in the current ruling market hegemony human need is seen as despicable dependence. Continuing care has been moved from long-stay hospital wards into the fragmented private sector with no obviously better results. Need and dependence in the young is seen differently. Value is put on the lives of children whose potential may be seen sentimentally, containing the seeds of what is to come. Older people are valued less. They are seen as having lost youth rather than gained experience. We contrast in identities the becoming self of childhood with the unbecoming self of old age. Zoja (1983) lists the expropriation of the traditional roles of older people – wisdom by the professionals; story telling by the media; holding the memories by computer.

With an ageing population, i.e. one with few younger people, a different ageism may be emerging. Older people with pensions are seen as a good target for consumer advertising and exploitation. With pension funds failing and the number of retired people increasing, social policies about age are a thinly veiled economic argument purporting to encourage older people to make a valuable contribution. This is by remaining in work. People should be discouraged from retiring as it is too expensive. The old ageism saw old people as dependent, the new ageism is about making them work (Biggs 2003) instead of allowing the space needed for attention to spirituality, integration and the changing self in old age.

The notion of change in adult life while usually associated with ideas of decline (unless we want older people to work) has another perspective. Cicero (45 BC) writes a clear evocation of the positive changes which old age may bring: 'It is not by muscle speed or physical dexterity that great things are achieved, but by reflection, force of character and judgement; in these qualities old age is usually not only not poorer but is even richer'. It is probably not helpful to merely counter arguments which denigrate with those which idealise old age (Garner and Ardern 1998). Some psychoanalysts eschewing Freud's opinion of the limit to development after adolescence have seen the possibility for psychological growth throughout life; some individuals achieve this progress more easily than others. Jung (1931) was the first adult developmentalist. He wrote of life having a 'morning' and an 'afternoon' with different principles governing each. The wise old man will discover a new focus in his internal world, away from the external (Bacelle 2004). Erikson (1959), a professor of human development at Harvard University, saw development extending throughout the lifecycle with specific psychosocial tasks to be negotiated during the eight phases he described. The phase specific conflict requiring internal mediation in old age, while also building on previous stages, is between 'Ego Integrity and Despair'. Those who possess integrity in old age see their life, their position in the world and in history, to be as it had to be. It was the right life for them, the right identity. Those without this emotional integration feel despairing that life is now coming to an end, there is no time to take a different path through life, they fear the inevitable 'not being' rather than taking satisfaction and valuing 'having been'. Other psychoanalysts have acknowledged the development that continues into old age and have delineated the social and psychological difficulties to be overcome in this process (Garner 2004). The pluripotentiality of the child inevitably becomes more restricted over the years but if things go well, for the individual psychologically, taking whatever walk is laid out through life, at the end the canvas will feel complete and as it should have been.

However well individuals may deal with the exigencies and difficulties of old age, wider society continues to view old age in terms of stereotypes, 'the dirty old man', 'the sweet old lady', 'there is no fool like an old fool'. Old age is a time of multiple losses and is often characterised as absences: absence of youth, absence of attractiveness, absence of sexuality, absence of productivity and finally absence of mind. A dementing illness is the caricature of old age and thought to be synonomous with it although 75 per cent of people over 80 do not have a dementia. The diagnosis is poorly understood outside of the health service and not always there. The word demented in common usage signifies being out of one's mind, being crazy, having lost touch with reality. The Alzheimer's Society, a charity established to promote the interests and support of those with Alzheimer's disease and of their families has a good press and has achieved much in advertising the disease and advocating on behalf of sufferers but still there is confusion. Patients' relatives often say something like 'I am prepared to hear it is senile dementia but please don't tell me it is Alzheimer's disease' or vice versa. Those with a different dementia, e.g. vascular, Lewy Body, frontotemporal, etc. may rather wish to be diagnosed with Alzheimer's disease and therefore to join that grouping with its articulate spokespeople.

Alzheimer's disease: identity and the patient

Alois Alzheimer described this condition in 1907 in a woman of 57. It is now recognised as the most common of the primary dementing illnesses. It is essentially a neuropathological diagnosis which can only be confirmed post mortem. A full history, examination of the mental state, physical investigations and psychometric testing point fairly conclusively to the diagnosis in life. The clinical picture is characterised by a global impairment of functioning affecting intellect, memory, language, skills, personality, affect, behaviour and sense of self. The disease is progressive, there are no treatments which cure although biological, psychological and social interventions have all been shown to temporarily reduce the progression for some patients. The overt signs – dysmnesias, dysphasias, dyspraxias, disabilities and discontents – are easy to describe. It is less simple to understand the experience of the one to whom this is happening. A few have written of their experience as have some family members but these are exceptions. The only way for others to come anywhere near an understanding of what it may feel like is by close and empathic listening to the patient, an understanding of the countertransference and that by projective identification the patient will give you some version of his experience even when speech is failing; unable to speak, the patient may still be riven by extreme emotional states (Wadell 2000).

In the initial stages, he is apparently more egocentric, withdrawing from others and not wanting social encounters. He may project his unacceptable feelings and blame others for his difficulties. In an attempt to hold on, during what feels like personal disintegration, previous character traits may become emphasised: the obsessional man more rigid; the quarrelsome one more aggressive. The disease feels like an attack on the self. There is a sense that the self is being lost along with all the other losses occasioned by the condition. The patient feels an existential terror, a sense of being abandoned in the world, or is it the world which is collapsing, ontological security is crumbling. Fear of abandonment and inability to bear separateness are familiar to all at some time but these persecutory states of mind increase many-fold with increasing organic impairment (Waddell 2000). The patient may follow his wife incessantly round the house not letting her out of his sight. The energy expended in needing to hold onto the self leaves little left to attend to the needs of others (O'Connor 1993) and the egocentricity may grow. There is a feeling of being uncontained and out of control. Catastrophic reactions sometimes occur when the anxiety is too great to be defended against; for Kohut (1972) this is a 'narcissistic rage' against the shame and humiliation regarding a defect in the self. Those who have erected a false self (Winnicott 1960) for the protection of the true self already have great difficulty coming to terms with old age and the loss of props to self-esteem, their plight is worse in the dementing process as skills in the carapace of the structured self are lost.

The fear with Alzheimer's disease is that one loses individuality and self-hood. Harris and Sterin (1999) looked qualitatively at the definition and presentation of the self in individuals with the early stage of the disease. They found a sense of losing the self. A loss of roles which had bolstered the sense of self and emotional reactions linked to efforts to maintain it. Core values of self-identity were meaningful productivity, primacy of autonomy and importance of comfort and security. Gil *et al.* (2001) examined various aspects of self-consciousness in Alzheimer's disease. The least disturbed aspects were mental representation of the body and awareness of identity. Capacity for introspection was not related to the severity of dementia and consciousness of identity remained regardless of cognitive test score. Tappan *et al.* (1999) looked at nursing home residents in the middle and late stages of Alzheimer's disease using conversation analysis. Residents coherently and frequently used the first person pronoun suggesting to the authors that awareness of self persists into severe Alzheimer's disease.

In the later stages of the disease, some develop autoprosopagnosia, an inability to recognise oneself in the mirror. This is not usually distressing and the patient may develop a relationship with 'that nice man'. Rarely the reduplicative syndrome of subjective doubles (Christodoulou 1978) may occur in which there is the belief that the self has been doubled. As the disease progresses to the final stages, the use of indexical pronouns breaks down. Do these phenomena indicate that the self, the identity, the person, has been lost? Does the concept of a unified self, the intuitive 'I am' break down in dementia? Perhaps the self remains there but hidden and imprisoned, unable to interact with the outside world. Can I know that 'I am' without knowing 'what I am'? 'Cogito, ergo sum': 'I think, therefore I am', Descartes' phrase, known to all schoolchildren, may actually limit our understanding of people with dementia. The patient may expand the idea for us. Bodily memories, skills, preferences, relationships do not deteriorate to the extent that higher thinking does. Affectivity is retained long after thinking is impaired; rituals and movement may prompt some recall, the ability to recognise far outlasts the ability to recall. He may be able to remember limited aspects of his autobiography long after he has ceased to be able to update it, sense of gender may continue to be a source of self knowledge, identity and even gratification well beyond the ability to say 'I am a man' is lost. Language is not the whole of our internal experience, an emotional life may continue unverbalised. For those who can tolerate dependency, the comfort and security of having bodily needs attended to may help define the self by containing anxiety. The self is not lost although there is little control over personal identity.

Advance directives written when someone had capacity to make choices and decisions to inform a time when they would be unable, perhaps by virtue of being unconscious, raise particular issues in a discussion of identity and Alzheimer's disease. If the patient with dementia no longer remembers the self who wrote the advance directive should notice be taken of it in regard to the treatment of this current self. Is the change over time a loss of self or merely a loss of capacity, the anticipated reason for writing the directive in the first place? It could be a tool for prolonging the individual's autonomy in dementia. The discussion about whether it is the same self or person over time does not particularly help in the clinical situation. That he is a person is what makes this work and decisions about end-of-life care so difficult (Hughes 2001). The advance directive requires acknowledgement. It should be talked about, it does not have to be acted on. It is an instrument not an instruction, part of the life story to be integrated into the present-day dialogue about the patient.

Some social constructionist considerations

Social constructionism is the analysis of 'reality' as contingent upon social relations. People actively construct their and others' social world. Dementia may be understood in biological and cognitive reductionistic terms – damage to this area of brain produces this disability; the representation of this word is matched with a representation of this meaning. Discursive psychology is anti-reductionistic. It does not look into the brain, rather it uses a social constructionist account of meaning which is not encoded in the head but in the conversation. Meanings are constituted by social interaction, by what occurs next in the conversation. We could no longer be subject and observer but co-workers remaking our world. The chapter author, a doctor, is aware of speaking about 'the patient' while reading accounts by others who write of the individual or sufferer with Alzheimer's disease. 'Patient' is a respected and respectful word, etymologically 'one who is suffering or enduring'. Nevertheless it positions the patient and the doctor differently. This is acceptable. Within the power dynamics of their asymmetric relationship, 'the doctor' as doctor will have access to investigative or management systems and skills which may be helpful. The patient's presentation of self needs to be seen in this context. The problem would be if the person was seen only as a patient and the doctor behaved only as a doctor.

Gollander and Raz (1996) describe the construction of social identity in an institution. Patients with Alzheimer's disease were labelled with their former social identities by non-cognitively impaired residents. Actual intentions of the residents with dementia were of less relevance than their social interpretation. Biographical fragments were socially re-edited; she was 'the knitter', 'the cook', 'the teacher' and enlarged into a personality leitmotif. The social construction of the 'demented role' by non-cognitively impaired residents involved a degree of scapegoating but also some envy of the one with dementia who could behave as they liked but with some good excuse, no pressure to get well and the benefit of not knowing the state they were in; they had a certain freedom being exempted from responsibilities and obligations; dementia: the blessing and the curse.

Sabat and Harre (1992) examine the loss of self in dementia from a social constructionist view of the nature of the self. This is expanded by Sabat *et al.* (1999) and Sabat (2001). Starting with the approach that personal self exists behind the publicly presented repertoire of one's personae, they show that there is a personal singularity that remains intact despite the disease even in the most debilitating stages. It is other aspects of the person that are socially and publicly presented that can be lost but then only indirectly as a result of the disease, rather due to the ways others react to the patient. The patient is positioned as helpless and confused, all behaviour is understood in relation to this positioning. The way people behave towards the individual with dementia will influence the way he behaves. 'Self One' is the self of personal identity, that singular point of view from which each person perceives the world and which remains with dementia. 'Self Two' is the self of mental and physical attributes both current and throughout life. At the present time with dementia one may have dysfunctional attributes as well as knowledge of previous qualities and attributes – having benefited from a good education, having a good memory, having a diagnosis of Alzheimer's disease. Frustration, anger, sadness seen as symptoms of the disease are reactions to 'Self Two' attributes, the social situation in which the patient finds himself and the way he is treated. Everything may be seen as part of the diagnosis – if the patient is angry about his difficulties it is a symptom, if he is not then he is apathetic which is a symptom. 'Self Three' comprises the plethora of social personae which are constructed with the co-operation of others: loving spouse, respectful child, devoted friend, admired teacher, etc. With Alzheimer's disease it becomes more difficult to enlist the co-operation of others. The only persona others may allow is that of patient with a diagnosis and a focus on his defects. This way of conceptualising self with its implications for improved communication and management for supporting selfhood is in line with the work of Tom Kitwood. Persons with Alzheimer's disease are persons behaving like persons.

Alzheimer's disease: identity and the family

'Who is it that can tell me who I am?' cries King Lear (I: iv) on his way to personal and familial exile. Self-identity and its expression originates in the early dyadic relationship, the infant seeing himself reflected in mother's eyes (Winnicott 1967). Families continue to influence and shape identity and the way it is expressed, sometimes quite overtly ascribing identities 'she's the clever one, he's the sociable one'. Aspects of identity change as roles change through life: being half of a couple is different from being single – the newly-wed saying 'this is my wife' adds a conversational and social construction to a personal experience. The philosopher's paradoxical joke 'I did not have adultery with your wife because she is not the woman you married' is less amusing to the spouse of a patient with Alzheimer's disease who knows she has a husband but also knows it is not the man she married. The subtle early changes in the disease process may only be detected by someone who is intimate. Minor dysfunctions are added to the 'Self Two' attributes as are emotional reactions to changes which are perceived by the patient himself. Over time as losses mount for the patient they do also for the partner. Memories and images of oneself held in and by the person with dementia are being lost (Garner 1997) and then comes the pain of not being recognised by a spouse or by a parent, 'he does not know who I am'.

The patient with dementia presents increased dependency needs. Many documents write of 'patients and carers' as if they had one identity with needs and wishes which coincided. This is not the case. The respite care which may seem appropriate to give the carer a break may feel quite unacceptable to the patient. Within social policy documents a frequent discourse is that of 'the family' positioned as providing care. This locates family carers as powerful and the recipient of care as passive (Adams 2000). Opie (1992) describes three positions, all familiar to clinicians, relating to the process by which family members take on the identity of a carer. The carer's identity may emerge within the context of a long and positive relationship; or care may be taken on due to feelings of obligation and duty; or identity of carer is taken on with feelings of immense resentment and anger. Couples and families react and behave differently depending on their personal and relationship experience and histories. For many there are negative connotations of dependency and shifts in power relationships, but for some the changing roles may in part be an opportunity to renegotiate relationships in a positive and reparative way.

The couple may turn in on itself becoming more exclusive and emotionally interdependent. Partners may either undermine or support efforts at face saving as they may be involved in interpreting between the patient and the outside world. Some family members come to see themselves as the 'expert carer', others 'the failure'. The diagnosis has been used as a reason to separate after a difficult marriage; it may not be acceptable to leave your husband of forty or fifty years, more acceptable to have him put in a home because of his illness although others with a similar level of difficulties continue to live in their own houses. The patient may allow the partner to take over more tasks than necessary if within their relationship it is seen as helpful to construct the partner as the carer; or the partner may take over not with the agreement of the patient but because of their own needs: impatience, embarrassment for the patient and inability to tolerate the situation. Couple identity tends to decrease with increased care-giving;

the partner who helped you with problems now presents the problem and will have less skills to deal with it.

Skaff and Pearlin (1992) assumed that long term care-giving would affect and reshape the self-concept of the carer because profound changes in the organisation of peoples' lives are demanded in this role. They may no longer engage in previous activities, social involvement or employment. There is less contact with family and friends. As role engulfment occurs the carer is left with fewer sources of self-evaluation and the carer, having less varied sources of feedback, is more vulnerable to self-loss. The only identity left may be that of 'carer'. In Skaff and Pearlin's study, this happened more to spouses than to children, more to younger carers and more to women. Men approached the care-giving as a new employment; for women it added more domestic tasks to their existing ones but reduced their social contacts. Decreasing social contacts predicted increasing sense of self-loss. It can be seen that those family carers who involve themselves in local voluntary bodies or support groupings do benefit in terms of social contacts but also in creating a new role for themselves despite having lost an aspect of self in, for example, anticipated retirement plans.

Cohen-Mansfield *et al.* (2000), in looking at self identity in people living in a nursing home suffering from dementia, found that the activities most likely to enhance the sense of identity was going for a walk and having family visits. The familial role was the most coherent identity during dementia but frequently it was the role in the family of origin as if it were their present reality. The patient with a moderate dementia often believes his parents are alive. Miesen (1993) has termed this 'parent fixation' and sees it not as a dysmnesic problem but as an equivalent of attachment behaviour in response to the fear and feeling of loss evoked by the disease.

MacRae (2002) writes of 'identity maintenance work' of the family members of the person with Alzheimer's disease. Although some family members see the patient as 'already gone', others cling on to the 'old self': 'she's still the woman she was', etc. Some developed ways of protecting the patient's social and self identity by covering up the memory loss, keeping the diagnosis a secret, blaming the disease not the person, making excuses, managing the appearance of the patient, recognising the self in touch, smile, a look in the eye. Families differed, some saw continuity in the dementia sufferer, others did not, perhaps as a reflection of their previous relationship and intimacy. The reluctance of some and wish of others to place someone in care may have something to do with whether or not continuity of self is seen.

Alzheimer's disease: identity and professionals

Staff bring the same prejudices and inner fears about old age and dementia as exist in the society of which they are a part. In the way that the patients are doubly stigmatised for being both old and mentally ill, so too by association are the staff who work with them. Alzheimer's disease has no cure and so threatens a doctor's and a nurse's identity as a professional, an identity which may have been incorporated into their idea of themselves as a person. The patients and staff may both feel the same fear of a loss of identity but staff are able to distance themselves from this by making an 'us and them' split between themselves and those for whom they are caring. Although the staff may fear they are seeing their projected self in old age, they can distance themselves from this by 'clinical detachment' which easily turns into emotional detachment and mindlessness (Terry 1997), finding it easier to do things to patients rather than engaging with them. In losing skills and independence it is easy to be seen no longer as a proper adult but to be infantilised, further emphasising the 'us and them' division; this may be in attitudes, in giving patients inappropriate clothes or hair ribbons or in the tone of voice and mode of address. Williams *et al.* (2003) looked at the way staff in nursing homes frequently communicate messages of dependence, incompetence and control to residents by using 'elderspeak'. This is a communication using diminutive endearments and inappropriate collective pronouns 'are we ready for our bath?' Staff use the first person plural in an attempt to get the patient to co-operate, i.e. using it to be instrumental rather than interactional (Smalls *et al.* 1998) but this can be infantalising and patronising. Identity is enmeshed in one's name. The denotation 'that is me' and connotation 'that sort of me' are inextricable from one's name. Being able to recall one's forename is likely to be the skill that remains longest. The patient should be asked how they wished to be called. Initially they may prefer to be known by their surname and a formal title, later they may be more comfortable with a forename or longstanding nickname. Each individual will be different.

People enter the health service and caring professions wishing to help patients. We want them to get better. When they do not, this may engender feelings of aggression, sadism, anxiety, guilt or depression. The patient may get the sedative when the staff can no longer tolerate the patient's continuing problems rather than for his direct benefit (Main 1957). The potential for abuse of these vulnerable patients is enormous particularly if they are construed as not being fully persons, having lost personhood. Within the staff, different groups have rather different identities and it is easy for further 'us and them' divisions to occur, e.g. those who call into the ward for visits, the doctor, psychologist, social worker, may see themselves as 'expert', knowing how patients should really be treated whereas the actual eight-hour shift of heavy physical work with the expectation of sensitive psychosocial skills in addition, is left to the more poorly paid nurses and care assistants. Identities along the continuum powerful to powerless exist throughout the institution. The least powerful staff are nevertheless in a position above the patients. In the way that behaviour labelled 'problem' in the patient may be an attempt by them to take some control over their life, so too may staff powerlessness within the institutional hierarchy be acted out in ill treatment of the patient (Garner and Evans 2001).

Staff may not be remembered to be named by patients at the level of cognitive skill but they are recognised and responded to affectively. Staff elicit different and consistent reactions. At some level, the patient knows that this is the one who is warm and comforting and understands me but this is the one who annoys, disturbs and upsets me. Something or someone is recognised in the staff and that needs to be reciprocated by them. If it is borne in mind that personal identity persists despite Alzheimer's disease, there will be a less task orientated approach to work. Patients will be more able to respond appropriately and co-operatively if they are treated personally, as themselves with preferences and idiosyncrasies preserved. A complex view of autonomy and capacity should be taken. Autonomy may be retained for some types of decision while being lost for others. It is difficult communicating with someone with a confusional state; staff need to be skilled in maximising their own understanding and the capacity of the patient. Even patients with significant impairment are able to make choices about their lives and environment. Staff have a role in supporting and preserving self-hood; in treating the patient as a gendered being: a witty man, a glamorous woman, a respected lawyer, etc. In order to do this well, they need as much information as possible from the patient themselves and from collateral sources. Reminiscence work assists in maintaining a narrative identity. Life history books help both the patient and relatives who will have a contribution to make. The physical environment with familiar artefacts and activities could be a therapeutic resource to encourage autonomy, to trigger reminiscence and a sense of continuity of the self. Cohen and Weisman (1990) write of encouraging 'wandering', not a problem to be controlled but independent mobility and an opportunity to engage in activities en route.

Researchers in the field of Alzheimer's disease tend to be fairly clearly split into those looking into the brain for a cause and a cure and those who look at the person not the disease. Both approaches are necessary. The medical view of dementia with its emphasis on accurate diagnosis is essential so as not to miss a potentially reversible cause of confusion. Having made the diagnosis, it needs to be remembered that this is not in the abstract: there is a person with the illness. Recent work (Gabbard 2000) indicating neurobiological changes associated with psychotherapy suggests the possibility of an integration of the two approaches. Patients with dementia could only benefit from this.

Cultural perspectives, identity, ageing and Alzheimer's disease

We draw on memories to construct stories about ourselves to retain and validate our self-identity and personal narrative. We do this in a psychosocial context which also involves religion, ethnicity and culture. Those with a cultural heritage distinct from the majority population will have a different narrative and may have a different experience of old age and dementia. Waid and Frazier (2001) in Florida, USA, found Hispanic elders were more likely to report family-related selves; Caucasian elders more likely to report selves in the abilities/education, physical and cognitive domains. Hinton and Levkoff (1999) in a qualitative study of different groups of caregivers in Boston, USA, found a subset of Chinese care givers narrating stories which emphasised how families managed confusion and disabilities; how they had or had not lived up to filial responsibilities; the changes were ultimately construed as an expected part of growing old and so were seen with less trepidation. A subset of Puerto Rican and Dominican families placed the elder's illness in stories of tragic losses, loneliness and family responsibility – perhaps caused by the death of a child or a spouse. In each type of story biomedical and folk understandings of Alzheimer's disease are combined.

Dementia affects members of all cultural groups. There is a convenient idea that some communities 'look after their own'. Convenient because then we have less obligation to provide appropriate and culturally sensitive services. Those who work with older people in the West have looked with admiration to the East where our image is of older people having a special and revered place; advancing age has been a cause for celebration, filial piety, respect and deference. However, with increased globalisation of materialism, the Confucian ideal of honouring and cherishing the old may be becoming obscured by the trappings and insistence of modernism. In modern Japanese literature (Loughman 1991) the Confucian ideal has been challenged by writers who have called attention to the growing numbers of elderly and the personal and social problems of caring for them.

Patel and Prince (2001), using a qualitative study of focus groups in Goa, India, found that vignettes of dementia were widely recognised but it was not thought to constitute a mental health problem requiring medical care. Rather it was construed as a normal part of ageing. Dementia was recognised by community health workers but it was attributed to abuse, neglect or lack of love by the children. The family system of care seems to have been less reliable than had been claimed and was often conditional on the expectation of inheritance. Traditionally elders have been venerated in this society and the majority continue to live at home and are well cared for but perhaps because of increasing pressures on families there are more incidences of abuse and neglect. Shaji et al. (2003) in a qualitative study of care givers in Kerala, India, found that care was most often the responsibility of women (daughters-in-law) in the family. Despite high levels of education and literacy, little was known about the illness. Findings from the study closely paralleled clinical experience in the UK; looking after someone with Alzheimer's disease is associated with financial disadvantage and deterioration in mental health; the main sources of care giver strain are behavioural problems and incontinence as well as criticism from and disputes with other family members and lack of support from the health service.

Basting (2003) writes that the fear of Alzheimer's disease permeates the American cultural consciousness as an economic and personal worry.

Conclusion

Understandings of identity are a mosaic of ideas. The self is a complex, multi-layered entity of many components including awareness of past, present and future, physical, cognitive, emotional, relational, spiritual, socio-cultural aspects. It also comprises private and public parts. Identity may be an intellectual and sophisticated concept brought to mind when thinking of the nature of other people. With regards to ourselves, the first thought is the basic 'I am', me, myself, mine, the knowledge of existence. With further thought one elaborates further layers of identity but underlying it all is the basic 'I' or 'I am'. The additional layers will evolve over the years. In healthy old age, one has a more developed sense of self, more knowledge of 'who I am' having experienced decades of both the inner and outer world and their relationship.

Post-modern discontinuities, absence of structure and rapidity of change in society with concomitant chaos and confusion may mirror widely the problems of the patient with Alzheimer's disease who feels his world is collapsing and his self disintegrating. Dementia is dually constituted of psychobiological pathologies and social processes beyond the individual with the disease. Concentration solely on biomedical models of pathology will miss relational aspects of the self. There is a concentration on and excitement engendered by recently marketed anti-dementia drugs. People with Alzheimer's disease should not be denied any medical advances but there are no pressure groups to lobby for increasing provision of psychological and social therapies which will be as beneficial as current medication in the management of dementia and the maintenance of the self. People with dementia may have changes in the most individual aspects of personality which explains the devastating sense of loss in the intimate other. They may not be exactly the same person having lost many skills and gained dysfunctions but they are still a person. Health service staff and others meeting this person could think further in helping them retain more of selfhood in relationships, conversation, activities and design of surroundings.

Thinking that personhood is extinct gives rise to many social and ethical problems. There can be no line between those living humans who are persons and those who are not, although the history of the world is too often a tragedy where these distinctions have been made. The essential self, the singular self, is not lost in dementia but the extra coverings of self, the personae which have been constructed and which we use to ease our psychological and social passage through life have been assaulted and need support. Despite not thinking well with a dementing illness or even thinking at all nevertheless 'I am' until I die.

Acknowledgements

There was a joint conference between the Philosophy Special Interest Group and the Faculty of Old Age Psychiatry of the Royal College of Psychiatrists in Newcastle, Autumn 2002. Ideas from that conference have stayed in my mind and influenced this chapter, as have discussions with Dr. Lorenzo Bacelle.

References

Adams T. (2000) 'The discursive construction of identity by community psychiatric nurses and family members caring for people with dementia', *Journal of Advanced Nursing*, 32(4), 791–8.

Bacelle L. (2004) 'On becoming an old man: Jung and others' (Chapter 3) in S. Evans and J. Garner (eds) *Talking over the years. A Handbook of Psychoanalytic Psychotherapy with Older People,* London, Brunner-Routledge (in press).

Basting A. (2003) 'Looking back from loss: views of the self in Alzheimer's disease', *Journal of Aging Studies*, 17, 87–99.

Bell D. (1996) 'Primitive mind of state', *Psychoanalytic Psychotherapy*, 10, 1, 45–57.

Berezin M.A. (1972) 'Psychodynamic considerations of ageing and the aged: an overview', *American Journal of Psychiatry*, 128, 1483–91.

Biggs S. (2003) Talk at the London Centre for Psychotherapy, 21 June 2003.

Christodoulou G.N. (1978) 'Syndrome of subjective doubles', *American Journal of Psychiatry*, 135, 249–51.

Cicero M.T. (45 BC) '*De Senectute*' trans. W.A. Falconer (1923) *On old age*, Harvard University Press.

Cohen N. and Weisman G.D. (1990) 'Experimental design to maximise autonomy for older adults with cognitive impairments', *American Society on Aging*, US, vol. 14 (supplement), 75–8.

Cohen-Mansfield J, Golander H. and Arnheim G. (2000) 'Self identity in older persons suffering from dementia: preliminary results', *Social Science and Medicine*, 51,381–94.

Erikson E. (1959) 'Identity and the lifecycle. Psychological issues', monograph, International Universities Press. No. 1, New York.

Evans S. (1998) 'Beyond the mirror: a group analytic exploration of late life and depression', *Ageing and Mental Health*, 2, 94–9.

Gabbard G.O. (2000) 'A neurobiologically informed perspective on psychotherapy', *British Journal of Psychiatry*, 177, 117–22.

Garner J. (1997) 'Dementia: an Intimate Death', *British Journal of Medical Psychology*, 70, 177–84.

Garner J. (2002) 'Psychodynamic work and Older Adults', *Advances in Psychiatric Treatment*, 8, 128–37.

Garner J. (2004) 'Growing into Old Age: Erikson and others' (Chapter 6) in S. Evans and J. Garner (eds) *London Talking over the Years. A Handbook of Psychoanalytic Psychotherapy with Older People*, Brunner-Routledge (in press).

Garner J. (2004) 'Dementia' (Chapter 15) in S. Evans and J. Garner (eds) *Talking over the Years. A Handbook of Psychodynamic Psychotherapy with Older People*, London, Brunner-Routledge (in press).

Garner J. and Ardern M. (1998) 'Reflections on Old Age', *Ageing and Mental Health*, 2, 92–3.

Garner J. and Evans S. (2001) 'Institutional abuse of older adults', CR84, Royal College of Psychiatrists.

Gil R., Arroyo-Anllo E.M., Ingrand P., Gil M., Nean J.P., Ornon C. and Bonnand V. (2001) 'Self-consciousness and Alzheimer's disease', *Acta Neurologica Scandinavica*, vol 1, 104(5), 296–300.

Goffman E. (1959) *The presentation of self in everyday life*, Garden City, New York, Doubleday Anchor.

Golander H. and Raz A.E. (1996) 'The mask of dementia: images of demented residents in a nursing ward', *Ageing and Society*, 16, 269–85.

Harris P.B. and Sterin G.J. (1999) 'Insider's perspective: definity and preserving the self of dementia', *Journal of Mental Health and Aging*, 5, 3, 241–56.

Health Advisory Service (1985) *The Rising Tide*, HMSO.

Hinton W.L. and Levkoff S. (1999) 'Constructing Alzheimer's: narratives of lost identities, confusion and loneliness in old age', *Culture, Medicine and Psychiatry*, 23, 453–75.

Hughes J. (2001) 'Views of the person with dementia', *Journal of Medical Ethics*, 27, 86–91.

Hume D. (1739) 'A treatise of human nature' (Section VI, 300–12) in D.G.C. Macnabb (ed.) (1962) *Personal Identity*, Glasgow, Fontana/Collins.

Jung C.G. (1931) The stages of life. *Collected Works*, 8, 387–403.

Kohut H. (1972) *Self psychology and humanities*, London, Penguin.

Locke J. (1690) 'An essay concerning human understanding' (Chapter XXVI, 206–20) in A.D. Woosley (ed.) *Identity and Diversity*, Glasgow, William Collins (Fontana 1964.)

Loughman C. (1991) 'The twilight years: a Japanese view of aging. Time and Identity', *World Literature Today*, 65, 49–53.

Miesen B.M.L. (1993) 'Alzheimer's disease, the phenomenon of parent fixation and Bowlby's attachment theory', *International Journal of Geriatric Psychiatry*, 8, 147–53.

O'Connor D. (1993) 'The impact of dementia: a self psychological perspective', *Journal of Gerontological Social Work*, 20, (3/4), 113–28.

Opie A. (1992) *There's nobody there*, Oxford, Oxford University Press.

Parfit D. (1971) 'Personal identity', *Philosophical Review*, 80, 3–27.

Patel V. and Prince M. (2001) 'Ageing and mental health in a developing country: who cares? Qualitative Studies from Goa, India', *Psychological Medicine*, 31, 29–38.

Sabat S.R. (2001) 'Selfhood and the Alzheimer's disease sufferer' (Chapter 7) in *The Experience of Alzheimer's Disease. Through a Tangled Veil*, Oxford, Blackwell.

Sabat S.R. and Harre R. (1992) 'The construction and deconstruction of self in Alzheimer's disease', *Ageing and Society*, 12, 443–61.

Sabat S.R, Fath H., Moghaddam F.M. and Harre R. (1999) 'The maintenance of self esteem: lessons from the culture of Alzheimer's sufferers', *Culture and Psychology*, 5(1), 5–31.

Shaji K.S, Smitha K., Lal K.P. and Prince M.J. (2003) 'Caregivers of people with Alzheimer's disease: a qualitative study from the Indian 10/66 Dementia Research Network', *International Journal of Geriatric Psychiatry*, 18, 1–6.

Skaff M.M. and Pearlin L.I. (1992) 'Caregiving: role engulfment and the loss of self', *The Gerontologist*, 32, 5, 656–64.

Small J.A, Geldart K., Gutman G. and Scott M.A.C. (1998) 'The discourse of self in dementia', *Ageing and Society*, 18, 291–316.

Terry P. (1997) *Counselling the elderly and their carers*, Basingstoke, Macmillan.

Waddell M. (2000) 'Only connect: developmental issues from early to late life', *Psychoanalytic Psychotherapy*, 14, 3, 239–52.

Waid L.D. and Frazier L.D. (2001) 'Cultural differences in possible selves during later life', *Gerontologist*, 41, 191 Sp.Iss.

Wilde O. (1891) 'The picture of Dorian Gray', Oxford World Classic Paperback (1998), 23. Oxford, Oxford University Press.

William S.K, Kemper S. and Hummert M.L. (2003) 'Improving nursing home communication: an intervention to reduce "elder-speak"', *The Gerontologist*, 43, 2, 242–7.

Winnicott D.W. (1960) 'Egodistortion in terms of true and false self' in *The Maturational Processes and the Facilitating Environment*, London, Hogarth.

Winnicott D.W. (1967) 'Mirror-role of mother and family in child development' in *Playing and Reality*, 111–18, London, Tavistock (1971).

Zinkin L. (1983) 'Malignant mirroring', *Group Analysis*, XVI, 113–26.

Zoja L. (1983) 'Working against Dorian Gray: analysis and the old', *Journal of Analytical Psychology*, 28. 51–64.

5

The Irish in London: identity and health

David Kelleher and Greg Cahill

Introduction

The Irish are not only the largest immigrant group in London they have also been coming to England over a longer period of time than any other group. They still do not integrate very well into English society, however, and although some marry English partners and many spend their adult life working here, they still think of Ireland as home. The process of spending their lives in England yet thinking of themselves as Irish may mean that their identity is at times uncertain and this may in turn be an important contributory factor in explaining their poor state of both mental and physical health.

Before looking at the evidence for stating that the health of the Irish in England is poor, or looking at the processes involved in the construction of their identities, it might be useful to consider the process of emigration itself. The long history of emigration has meant that saying goodbye to family and the well-known local area and community has become part of the fabric of Irish society. Although for many it has been seen as being only short term, a period in which to earn some money, spread their wings for a while before coming home, it has become for many of them an unthinking permanent abode. It has also been one of the ways in which, through an unholy alliance of politicians and the Church, the holy Ireland of de Valera (Miller 1990; O'Connell 2001) continued as an underdeveloped pastoral economy until, that is, the seductive effects of EEC membership and the boom years of inward investment in the 1980s led to the 'Celtic tiger' of the 1990s, and to a reduction of emigration and even the return of many.

Most writers on the subject suggest there are several main reasons why people emigrate from Ireland. The first is either to find work or to seek a better job abroad. The next major reason is that they feel stifled in the family and community in which they are living and think that the world outside offers them adventure and a chance to develop. A third reason is to study and improve their educational qualifications. A small group of women leave because they are pregnant and not married. Several studies show the pattern of emigration and offer theoretical explanations: The Economic and Social Implications of Emigration (1991)(cited in Winston 2000) is an example of a government study which offers statistical detail but little enlightenment. A more interesting later publication (Winston 2000) draws on a sample of Irish people in London and on previous studies including previously unpublished material from one by the Economic and Social Research Institute (1991) (cited in Winston 2000) to identify some 'push' factors. These should be seen as going alongside the already mentioned factors. The 'push' factors she identifies are:

- people who were disillusioned with Ireland (e.g. those who viewed the system of taxation as 'punishing' and forcing them to leave);
- people fleeing situations of abuse (e.g. people, mainly women, who had experienced domestic violence);
- those who were forced to leave, such as those people from Northern Ireland expelled by paramilitary organisations or people from the Republic who had been involved in drugs and were compelled to leave by vigilantes.

(Winston 2000: 17)

A qualitative study carried out by the authors of this chapter (1997) supports and illustrates the main reasons referred to in the ESRI (1991) and the ESIE (1991) above. Only one or two people said they were forced to leave or were fleeing from what might be classed as abuse, including the one or two who said they had found life as a 'gay' person difficult in Ireland. The first respondent was one of four who illustrate the influence of the Catholic Church, the importance of being married and the harsh social treatment expected for becoming pregnant out wedlock:

> I left when I was just 16 and I was pregnant . . . Because my parents were Catholics and didn't actually know and I actually ran away.
>
> (young woman, interview 12)

An unemployed man said that he found the situation at home 'a bit too close'. He wanted to break out of the claustrophobic atmosphere and get a job. Another who had a good job in Ireland spelled out more precisely what was 'too close' for him as a gay man. If he had stayed in Ireland he would have:

> . . . been a closeted homosexual, a life of quiet desperation. I wouldn't be living at all but I would have learned how to survive in that society.
>
> (man in his 30s, interview 25)

A range of reasons for coming over were provided by another, but all of them related to her situation in Ireland:

> To look for work basically ... Well I had left Ireland with an honours leaving certificate and I hadn't qualified for a university place because, I plus I couldn't afford to pay for it, and secondly I had always wanted to be a teacher and unfortunately I failed to get the necessary qualifications in oral Irish.
>
> (woman in her 30s, interview 24)

She went on to say that she could not start a course in England straight away as she had to work to support a younger sister and brother in Ireland as her alcoholic father had 'done a runner' many years previously. An older man shared some of her reasons:

> I think it was natural leaving home, becoming independent thing any-way ... I left at 19 ... I did make some enquiries about going to college in Ireland and that didn't work out. My father was a teacher and he couldn't afford to pay the fees.
>
> (man in his 50s, interview 30)

Most of the others interviewed shared a similar range of reasons: looking for work and, as one young woman, said for 'a better way of life hopefully'; a sense of wanting to explore the big city; and to escape from the close control exercised by family and church in Ireland (an important reason for many of the younger people interviewed). Even a woman in her 50s, who came to England to start training as a nun, came because she said she felt nuns had a better time here, 'less strict' in England. Others came to continue their education, but a number of them came already well qualified. As this 50-year-old woman described:

> Well, I had been to university in Dublin, and I worked in Northern Ireland for a year in Social Services. And I felt there had to be a little bit more to life and looked for adventure.
>
> (interview 59)

MacLaughlin (2000) objects to the 'voluntaristic' kind of explanation which locates it at the level of individual choice and points to the structural reasons to do with Irish society and economy which are often conveniently not mentioned in official enquiries into the emigration problem, often preferring to talk of it as migration. This relates to the point made above by Miller and O'Connell, that many of those asked had no clear reason of their own but felt the cultural push created by political and economic leaders over time.

Walter (2001: 15) makes a related point in showing that one of the striking things about emigration from Ireland is that the numbers of women emigrating at most periods exceeded the numbers of men. They came to England, she suggests, for many of the same reasons as men but in addition she finds two further reasons: women were not able to inherit the family land; from 1923 until 1973 married women were not allowed to remain in most occupations. Only the introduction of EEC labour regulations forced the change in government policy then.

The experience of the Irish in England

One of the important factors which make the identity of Irish people in England problematic, and likely to influence their health status, is the nature of their experience in England. They are surprised that their sense of *difference* (Derrida) is so pervasive, so much a part of everyday life. This is what makes them very aware of being Irish, something they had taken for granted before. This sharpened awareness of their own country is accompanied by a heightening of the observations of how they are regarded here and this contributes to the overall sense of being different. This is a comment that emigrants from other countries have also noted about themselves. With the Irish it is not, as is the case with black and Asian people, that there is a difference in their appearance which is remarked on; it is when they speak that the first sign of difference is noticed, particularly if they say numbers such as 'tirty–tree' which immediately is found laughable or when they use an Irish way of phrasing something. Sometimes the accent is thought to be attractive but even this is to have their difference pointed out. This Hiberno-English shows the influence of Gaelic which remains in some pronunciation and linguistic structures.

Our respondents often remarked that after this language difference is commented on, being addressed as 'Paddy' follows, a form of address which, by failing to use their personal name, negates an important part of their personal identity. The 'Paddy' name was sometimes extended to Irish women. Some were content to accept this way of noting their difference, of being clearly identified as being members of a group not-English, and sharing the same characteristics as all other people in that group, even those who planted bombs.

One of the chief characteristics of that 'Paddy' group is made clear in the Irish jokes they hear. Walter quotes from Buckley to show what she sees as the significance of the 'Irish' joke:

> The joke is a very significant hinge in Irish-British relations because it is one of the few locations or moments when reference to Irishness rises to the surface of British discourse. Politically it matters because it simultaneously expresses and obscures racism, facilitating racist interaction

while with the same gesture exculpating it as mere fun. When directly addressed to an Irish person, it can constitute an invitation to social bonding which rests on an oblique, mutual awareness of the uneven power-relations which the Irish person is invited to accept.

(Buckley 1997: 101, cited in Walter 2000: 89)

The point about the invitation to social bonding is important in that it is clear that the role of Irish people in the jokes is to show the superiority of the English and the kind of role offered to the Irish, that of being the likeable clown or stage Irishman.

As indicated above, another situation which has often been projected on to Irish people is that of IRA supporter. Respondents in the survey conducted by the authors frequently mentioned that people at work said to them after an IRA bombing had been reported, 'Oh I see your lot were at it again last night'. One middle-aged woman said that after one explosion she had been amazed to find that her local butcher refused to serve her and, on another occasion, a taxi driver drove off when he heard her accent as she told him her destination. Some tried to avoid such situations by saying little on public transport, even when travelling with a friend, but one or two said that they had got into fights as their way of responding. A different response came from one man who said that he actually apologised to his boss after the Warrington bombing because, as he said, to some extent the ideology he believed in had some responsibility for it, even though he believed only in peaceful means. Such doubts about Irish people may still be occurring as BBC television (16 December 2002) still finds it necessary to broadcast warnings about IRA terrorist threats.

In many ways and on many days, something happened pointing them out as not English, creating the sense of difference they experienced. Some had reacted to these experiences by socialising mainly with other Irish people, thus trying to avoid confrontation but becoming more deliberately Irish as a result. Others tried to lessen their accent so that their difference was less noticeable and to seek out English friends, in a sense denying their Irishness, but even then conflicts sometimes arose. One woman, who had integrated to the extent of marrying an Englishman, recounted how, when she and her husband were having a meal with a group of friends, she was asked for her views on the IRA. She tried to deflect the question at first but after persistent questioning, she attempted to give what she thought was a considered and honest answer which took into account the historical situation. The questioner thought her answer was outrageous, as she had indicated what he took to be support for a terrorist organisation. Although she tried to keep cool, it ended with her leaving the group on her own with the questioner saying he didn't know how her husband could bear to be married to such a woman.

Identity in doubt: the part played by ethnicity

References to identity are numerous in newspapers and in academic writing. This is more than fashion; it is a reflection of changing political structures, increased migration, the effects of globalisation and the consequent disembedding and changes in work situations, all of which add to the importance of being able to establish a personal identity, all have effects on the degree of certainty with which people can describe themselves to themselves and present themselves to others. Identity though is not purely a self-constructed phenomena; agency is tempered by structure. This relates to the varied encounters people have at work or in social life when living in a cosmopolitan city like London as well as the historical relations between England and Ireland. These encounters may challenge identity instead of confirming it as meetings in the towns and villages where they grew up in Ireland did, and where there is an unstated sense of community. Giddens (1991) in commenting on this kind of effect writes of how the disembedding mechanisms 'which prise social relations free from the hold of specific locales ... transform the content and nature of day-to-day social life'. The process he describes seems to be common to all immigrants, including the Irish, who although they have travelled only a short distance in spatial terms may have come from a close-knit community where they were known and greeted by everyone they met, to a place where to walk down the street is to pass only strangers. Whilst at times they might come to revel in the freedom from family and church control, this could easily become loneliness and anxiety if they are so often marked out as different, and have to work to establish a personal identity. The strains are accentuated if they do not find work and friends or make contact with relations living in London. In the study we conducted, a man, now in his 50s but who came over when he was 17, remembers well the loneliness:

> It was an awful shock to the system, because I couldn't get over people not talking to you in the street ... I hated London, I just wanted to save enough money to go home. I just hated it. It's such a big city and I came from the country, it was very hard to adjust, you know.
>
> (interview 51)

A woman in her 40s, who came over 17 years earlier told a similar story:

> Dreadful. The loneliness, not knowing anybody, growing up in a town where you knew everybody, leaving it all behind and knowing there would be four or five people here. That was the worst thing, not seeing sisters, mother, father or anything but still hoping to make a go of it.
>
> (interview 53)

Ethnicity and identity: the part played by others

In his work on questions of cultural identity, Hall (1994) comments on how the relatively unchanging identities of people in pre-Enlightenment times became the constructed and often fragmented identities of late modernity, when post-modern culture puts so much stress on personal identity.

It is perhaps not surprising that many Irish immigrants coming to London from what was until recently a traditional society had difficulty in establishing a continuing sense of selfhood given that many of them were still teenagers when they first emigrated (Laughlin 2000). The problem though was experienced by most of our respondents as they encountered the almost daily 'hassles' of being made to feel different. As one young woman working in a pub said:

> When I say my name is Laura, they go 'Oh I thought you were called Biddies, Maureens and Maire', that type of thing.
>
> (interview 12)

Some were able to handle such challenges to their identity, being seen simply as one of an outgroup, but others felt it strongly and responded by saying:

> If a man calls me Paddy, I say my name is Niall, and I only tell him once. After that he gets a fuckin' belt.
>
> (interview 19)

An older man who had come to England as a schoolteacher found the continual mimicking of his accent by boys and one or two staff so irritating and disturbing that he gave up teaching after one year.

Singly, any one incident was maybe trivial, but the cumulative effect of these tensions, the Irish jokes, assumed association with IRA bombings, of comments about their speech, all pointing out that they were 'others' to the English, emphasised the ethnic aspect of identity. They made it 'difficult to keep a particular narrative going across time and space' (Giddens 1991: 54) to continue to think of themselves as the same person that they were in Ireland.

Another strand of the ethnic difference is the historic Catholic/Protestant animosity. Although most of our sample were not regular attenders at Mass, religion was likely to be to the fore at christenings, weddings and when parents were choosing a school for their children. One young woman marrying an English man reported that though her wedding was in the familiar setting of a Catholic church, the wedding celebration was spoiled by the clumsy humour of the English best man. In his speech he presented the bridegroom with a hard hat and a shovel as he said, 'you're joining an Irish family now'. Walter (2000: 87) believes that although 'anti-

Catholicism remains deeply embedded in British nationalisms', particularly in Scotland, she later suggests that it may be lessening as they are joined together as 'Christian' in the 2001 census question on religion. This may be an assumption in the 'official mind' only of course, and may be a source of irritation to those who still want to identify themselves as not just Christian but Roman Catholic as well.

The problem for Irish people in London is that whether they came to England simply for work or to develop as well and to expand their lives and themselves (whilst maintaining a sense of coherence and authenticity) (Kelleher and Hillier 1996), they found they were soon identified as 'Paddies' with only the characteristics of those attributed to the Irish as a group and as seen by the English. The jokes, the name of 'Paddy' applied to them all, sometimes irrespective of gender, and, as mentioned earlier, were experiences they all reported. They were expected to be not very intelligent, friendly, hard working, liking a drink and sometimes a fight, confined to the stereotype created by the English, the English 'other'. This applied to men and women, to those working on building sites, behind the bar in a pub and even to one who was training to be a chef who was called a Fenian bastard by the head chef. All this made the ethnic aspect of identity something they had to struggle with, whereas before, in Ireland, they were proud of their Irishness but not conscious of it all the time. In England their ethnicity was constantly being remarked on even when they were not being challenged about it. As one young woman said:

> I like it when people come into the pub and they can tell before I even speak. 'They say are you Irish? Because you look Irish.' That's nice.
>
> (interview 12)

Other aspects of identity

But being Irish was not necessarily what they wanted to be the dominant aspect of their identity; they were young men and women and sometimes had ideas, sometimes vague to be sure, of who else they might identify with and what else they might become. An example of someone who was prob-ably the person who least wanted to cling to his Irish identity and was annoyed by those who, in England, identified with everything Irish, said he thought of himself as London Irish and said of those who insisted on pointing up their differences from the English:

> Because [to those who cling to their Irishness] the Irish are a tragic race, because they have all this tragedy behind them. Famine, and the differ-ence is you didn't have this, you'se didn't have the famine, you'se are the oppressors, we are the oppressed, that's the difference.
>
> (interview 14)

He did say though that if he were watching England play football against a European team he would, like most of those interviewed, support anyone but England suggesting that his Irishness is still a strong part of his identity.

As already noted, many said they came to look for work, and expanded on this by saying 'to look for a better way of life, hopefully' or 'I felt there must be more to life'. The man who said he had given up teaching after one year of being made fun of because of his accent said that he was, in the late 60s, 'enthused by these ideas [comprehensive education, free health care], certainly by education for all, which wasn't actually a reality in Ireland at that stage'. Some came to extend their education, 'the main purpose was self-improvement'. Others were less precise but seeking change nevertheless, 'To get a different outlook on life', or 'Well, um, I don't know, just wanted a different life, decided I was 21 and was old enough to do my own thing'. Others were less 'pulled' and more 'pushed' as this young man stated, 'I left when I was 16. I left from . . . in South Kerry. I'm the sixth child, and half a twin, father was an alcoholic'.

The young men and women who left Ireland had varying fortunes: they acquired degrees, learned trades and some married. Others that we interviewed in hostels had been less successful and had spent some time living on the streets or had a bad back or other disability as a result of an accident at work: some of the many Irish who suffered accidents and then found that they were not covered by an insurance scheme. For some of those who became nurses, teachers or social workers though, they enthused about work, and their profession became a part of their identity.

Methodology employed in the study

The quota aimed for a sample of 80 people but became an achieved one of 75. It was made up of men and women according to housing type, with 20 in each category: home owner; privately rented; council or housing association rented; hostel or homeless (this last group being the most difficult to find). The sample was designed in this way to cross cut a number of variables: classes; those who might be established here long enough to buy a house; the young who were likely to be renting; and those often omitted from such studies, those in hostels and who had recently been sleeping rough. Men and women were approximately equal in number in the sample. All respondents were aged between 18 and 65 and had been in England for at least a year, with a number having been here for 20 to 35 years. While the sample size was smaller in number than most quantitative studies, the range of people included is probably greater, thus allowing for the possibility of analysis in greater depth.

Each respondent was interviewed for about an hour, using a non-standardised interview schedule to encourage them to speak freely. The questions covered a range of topics, including why they came to England, their experiences of work and other people, including how they thought Irish people were viewed, eating, smoking and drinking habits and any experiences they had of the English healthcare system. They were then asked to complete the SF 36 to assess their health status.

The interviews took place mainly in the respondent's home or in a room at their hostel; some took place in a pub if they worked there. All the interviews took place in situations where the respondents felt comfortable. Most interviews were carried out by Cahill, who is himself a Dubliner.

Theories of identity

As indicated earlier, Hall (1994) and other writers examine how the relatively unchanging identities of people in pre-Enlightenment times became the often fragmented sense of identity of the present in post-traditional modern society. The theories of writers as different as Marx, Habermas, Durkheim, Mead, Erikson, Giddens and Hall, to take a selection of the most important of them, all agree on the elements in the construction of identity but give differing importance to these elements: the individual mind, interaction with others, the degree of reflexivity and the structures of society.

The approach taken by Mead is clear in the title of his major work, *Mind, Self and Society*, in which he emphasises the relationship between these. Blumer makes this clear in his article 'Sociological implications of the thought of George Herbert Mead'.

Mead's concern was predominantly with symbolic interaction. Symbolic interaction involves interpretation, or ascertaining the meaning of the actions or remarks of the other person, and definition, or conveying indications to another person as to how he is to act (Blumer 1969: 66).

It is through this interaction and the reflexive process of the 'self', according to Mead, that identity is constructed; in this view it is through their interpretation of what they experience in England, that Irish people derive their view of themselves as seen by the English. As Mead makes clear though, how they are addressed and treated is a matter for them to interpret. For some the jokes are just banter, but for others when they are coupled with being given a group identity with the shared name of 'Paddy' and with insinuations being made of their involvement in terrorism, their sense of personhood is made fragile. As Mead, and later Giddens, have stressed, the construction of identity is made up not only of inputs from 'significant others' like workmates and the generalised 'other' in terms of societal influences from the media, but of what the 'reflexive self' makes of these actions.

While Hall also makes clear that identity is a construction in much the same way as Mead, he also considers the possibility of a person having multiple selves and stresses that historical situations have an influence. Rutherford, commenting on the work of Hall, notes:

> Each individual is the synthesis not only of existing relations but of
> the history of these relations ... in the intersection of our everyday
> lives with the economic and political relations of subordination and
> domination.
>
> (Rutherford 1990: 19)

A factor relevant to many Irish immigrants who come to England with an
almost innate sense of historical subordination.

For Hall, identity is also multi-faceted suggesting that identities are never
fixed, but vary from one setting to another as he suggests in the pun made by
the close juxtaposition of roots and routes, saying that we need to understand our routes. Although the contribution of Hall to understanding the
construction of identity is profound, it is perhaps, Habermas with his
emphasis on language, who allows us to see most clearly the links between
structural forces and the moral situation of Irish immigrants.

Habermas builds on the work of Mead and emphasises the important
role, and essentially social nature of language, in developing his concept
of communicative interaction and for this reason his may be the most useful
approach in the study of Irish immigrants. As noted earlier, they may experience their sense of difference when their language is commented on.
Habermas, in talking about communicative practice of different lifeworlds
notes:

> Traditional, habitual forms of life find their expression in particular
> group identities marked by particular traditions that overlap one
> another, compete with one another, and so on ...
>
> (Habermas 1987: 108)

He goes on to outline how the concrete, conventional ego-identity that
immigrants bring with them is 'cancelled, and preserved in a new synthesis'
as individuals' identities are challenged and 'partly disintegrated' as they
existentially attempt to work at who they want to be. This seems to be
the position of many of the subjects in our study; they find that the lifeworlds they inhabit are not shared by the English people they encounter,
their ways of understanding how to live and the assumptions made about
them do not help them to integrate into society. Habermas moves from
Mead's interpersonal level of analysis to considering how Durkheim leads
him on to developing his own more Marxist analysis which links communicative interaction to structural considerations.

He does this by indicating how the lifeworld, which is the basis from
which individuals unconsciously draw ideas of how to interact with others
and is the basis of integration, has become interpenetrated and increasingly
governed, 'colonised', by the instrumental rationality of capitalist society.
This form of rationality and the medium of money are the links Habermas

makes between system and lifeworld. In the lifeworld, people normally interact using the Meadian process of taking the role of the other and so integrating their acts together; but as noted above, Habermas adds his own stress on the importance of language in this process of communicative interaction. In the interactions between English people and Irish people, Irish people (as has been indicated in the earlier quotations) often have difficulties with taking the role of the other and in getting anywhere near the Habermasian ideal of an undistorted speech situation, the kind of situation in which by putting forward their views, speakers can reach agreement or clarify their positions; the assumption of all communicative interaction being that speakers desire to reach understanding. But to do this means that neither speaker uses power or influence to dominate the other, conditions which approach an ideal speech situation. But deconstructing the meaning of the Irish joke, and the situations commonly described by Irish people serving in bars or similar situations, shows that not only is their personal identity being denied them but the purpose of the language used by people talking to them is coercive (perlocutionary in the theory of language Habermas adopts from Austin). In these coercive exchanges, they are regarded as symbols and without an independent moral status, unable to take the role of the other as hypothesised in Meadian theory. In such situations they are reduced to wage-slaves, the medium of money linking system and lifeworld, any idea of self-realisation fades, the lives of many of those without degrees or a professional job become lives of drinking with mates in the warm companionship of the pub, dreaming of home, home being the Ireland of their memory and imagination. Even though those in professional jobs are able to afford to fly home more often, it is noteworthy that they still think of Ireland as home and may also telephone weekly to keep in touch. All of them still think of themselves as Irish but are irritated at being thought of as IRA supporters. As mentioned previously, such encounters led to many saying that they kept quiet with their heads down when travelling on buses and tube trains and in other public places.

The effect of such limitations in the public sphere, the link between the lifeworld and the power structures of society may explain the reluctance of the Irish in England, unlike in the USA, to organise themselves politically and this inability to draw strength from the collectivity perhaps contributed to the development of problematic identities. Kelleher and Hillier note:

> the sense of collective insecurity about their identity which may contribute both to their unwillingness to make demands on the healthcare system and to the likelihood that their problems may eventually emerge as psychological ones, or at least be diagnosed as such.
>
> (Kelleher and Hillier 1996: 121)

The health of the Irish in Britain

The argument now put forward is the reverse of that in most chapters where the writers have looked at the effects on identity of having a chronic illness; what is considered here is how the experience of living in England affects identity and how this in turn can be linked to the strikingly poor mental and physical health of Irish people in England. The evidence for their generally poor health has been apparent for some time and recent summaries show this to be continuing. Kelleher and Hillier (ibid) survey a range of evidence comparing the health of Irish people in England with the general population of England and Wales and also, on some measures, that of Irish emigrants with the population of those in Ireland, to show that the health of the Irish in England is 'significantly poorer' than that of the native English. Tilki uses some different data to reach the conclusion that 'Irish people living in Britain have significantly higher mortality rates...' (Tilki 1996: 11). Balajaran (1995) presents a similar picture across a range of conditions from coronary heart disease 75.5 per 100,000 (all Ireland place of birth) compared with native English 59.3; of other immigrant groups, only those from Bangladesh, Pakistan and India were higher. Irish people were higher than native English for deaths from strokes and lung cancer, although Irish women suffered fewer deaths from breast cancer than English women. The position of the Irish in England in relation to mental health is summarised in a paper by Bracken *et al.* in 1998. They say,

> Evidence that the Irish are grossly over-represented as users of psychiatric services has been available for a number of years.
>
> (Bracken *et al.* 1998: 172, 103–5)

They also comment on the excessively high rate of suicide amongst the Irish in England. This is taken up by Leavey (1999) who, in a detailed examination of suicide rates, concludes that not only is the suicide rate of Irish people in England higher than indigenous English people, but it is also higher than Irish people in living in Ireland. Interestingly he also links the high suicide rate to the problem Irish people in England have in establishing an authentic identity.

At the macro-social level, the Irish community has been disabled in achieving a distinct ethnic identity within Britain and, for understandable historical reasons, strongly resist the possibility of a British identity (Leavey 1999: 170).

The people in the study used as a basis for this chapter provide some examples of the lifestyles and concerns of Irish people in London across an age-range of 40 years. A professional man in his 40s and living in many ways happily with a partner admitted to bouts of homesickness and guilt about the daughter he had left in Ireland. He regularly drank with friends in the pub on four nights a week. Another younger man who shared a house with five other men had moved on from labouring to become a carpenter because,

> I just knew looking at the people around ... I don't want to end up like them ... bent backs and I knew where they got it from. It was definitely work because you could feel it in your back coming home.
>
> (man in his 30s, interview 14)

In getting a trade, he said he had improved his income but he was unhappy about the dusty environment he usually had to work in and about the food he had to eat in England because in Ireland the vegetables were fresher and the milk was better. He felt he drank less than he did in Ireland though, going to the pub only once during the week because he might have a date. At weekends though,

> We'll say from Friday night from finishing work through 'til closing time. Saturday, go to work in the morning, finish, go home but you'll only be going and washing and ready for 7 or 8 [o'clock] because you're going out and you're probably going to be on the pull so you want to look okay ... You go out all night – 3 o'clock in the morning, maybe 4 get home. Such a hangover next day that everybody goes to the pub. Sunday morning Irish ballad session.
>
> (man in his 30s, interview 14)

Overall, he said he would drink about 30 pints over the weekend. He would smoke 120 cigarettes. He also felt stressed, he said, because a previous relationship he had had [in England] resulted in the woman having a child although he had wanted her to have an abortion. But he was also stressed by:

> Trying to get a plan together. It's hard to know exactly what you want. It depends on how much you think about it ... It depends on how you view yourself. Whether you've succeeded in what you want over here or whether you've failed and where are you going. The usual question is what are you doing with your life. With the Irish culture they all ask each other the same questions.
>
> (man in his 30s, interview 14)

The women in the sample varied from the three who came because they were pregnant, and decided to keep their babies despite the difficulties of managing work and childcare while being still a young woman, to one who badly burned her hand working in a laundry but by working hard managed to get accountancy qualifications, to another who trained as a teacher but retired early because of back pain and stress. A young professional woman who came because she was pregnant said she found the first two years chaotic and still misses her family but now had a council house. She was stressed by financial worries, used a counsellor to off-load her worries and still tried to lead the life of a young woman:

> I walk in parks, drink, go to playgrounds, clubbing, reading and baths.
>
> (woman in her 20s, interview 20)

A young woman who worked as secretary found not only getting to work stressful, as many people living in London do, but found London itself 'a hostile place' and the pace of the work environment too fast:

> I find the office very stressful... I work with quite young people who are trying to get there very fast, trying to make money very fast...Work is their life whereas it isn't mine. It's part of my life but I don't find it's my be all and end all of everything.
>
> (woman in her 30s interview 72)

The older woman who trained as a teacher in England had had a variety of jobs first:

> I couldn't do that straight away because I left behind a younger sister and a brother who was very ill and an alcoholic father who had done a runner many years before that so the option for me was to work. I worked first of all for a while in Smiths factory and a variety of office jobs and I finally applied for the GPO. I was accepted ... worked there for 6 years ... met my husband ... had a baby daughter ... did a variety of jobs again ... In 1980 qualified as a primary school teacher ... worked there for 16 years ...The last three years though I damaged my knee and went to the doctor and he told me it was arthritis ... went back to school ... in excruciating pain and as a result damaged a nerve in my back.
>
> (woman in her 50s, interview 24)

She became very pressured at work despite pain, including by this stage a damaged retina, and so retired. The back was then diagnosed as a cyst on her spine. Another teacher in the sample also retired early with a bad back and 'an Irish health' as she described it.

The SF 36 results provided further supportive evidence of the health status of the sample. In the health perception section 78 per cent rated their overall health as only 'fair to good' and in the mental health section, the results showed that for men and women combined 89 per cent were below the mean, the mean being arrived at from English sample studies.

Linking identity and poor health

There is no one explanation for the overall burden of poor health of Irish people in England, but one factor which may contribute to their poor mental health may well be the kind of experiences described earlier, the sense of difference they are made to feel. The almost daily 'hassles' when their accent is remarked on or the malicious suggestion that they may be associated with the IRA that many people in our sample described are likely to have made identities precarious, the development of a 'continuing narrative' as Irish people a difficult task. At a common-sense level, this can be seen as most likely to affect their mental health and a number of writers develop this point. Kelleher and Hillier (1996) use the coherence theory of Antonovsky (1963) developed in relation to Jewish people and Sartre's concept of authenticity to relate it to the Irish in England. Antonovsky looked at the experience of Jews in America and suggested that

> The modern emancipated Jew does not know fully who he is, and much of what he does know he cannot accept. He is the stranger who does not wish to be a stranger... He retains the old label of Jew but has no identity acceptable to himself. It is this lack of an acceptable identity which is the core of the problem for the Jew.
>
> (Antonosky 1963: 428)

Leavey (ibid) in coming to his conclusion about the high suicide rate of the Irish in England also makes use of the concept of authenticity. This problem may also affect physical health.

The 'hassles' concept may be seen as a form of stress, itself an important concept about which there is a considerable literature but a variety of definitions. Delongis *et al.* (1982) found that daily hassles 'the repeated or chronic strains of everyday life' 'were more strongly associated with somatic health than were life-events scores'. Chamberlain and Zika (1990) argue that the more recent view of stress has been from the 'minor or everyday events' and that hassles are 'substantially better than life-events in predicting psychological well-being and mental health dimensions'. Steptoe (1991) notes that the links between stress and ill-health are poorly defined but goes on to make the important point that

> in terms of aetiology and maintenance of illness, the traditional distinctions between psychiatric disorders [and] physical disorders ... is outmoded. Rather, psychosocial factors may influence the entire spectrum of health disorders.
>
> (Steptoe, 1992: 633)

This is an important step in the argument which is sometimes despairingly acknowledged by general medical practitioners when treating an illness which is not responding to drug therapy. It is also important to recognise that individuals vary in their susceptibility to illness. A factor, which seems particularly relevant to Irish migrants, is the level of psychological and practical support which they feel they can draw on. Although most of those interviewed said they had someone to talk things over with, this was sometimes achieved by phoning 'home' and a number of young women said they missed having sisters and other family members to talk to.

Loneliness linked with the repeated and sometimes hostile hassles of being noticed as different may be linked in a general way to the kind of stress, which weakens the immune system. Kaplan (1991), reviewing a wide range of studies which consider the effects of such situations as bereavement, loneliness, 'negatively valued life-events, social identities [negatively valued identities] and ongoing strains in interpersonal relationships', concludes

> The literature on the whole strongly suggests that psychological factors have profound and complex influences on the functioning of the immune system.
>
> (Kaplan 1991: 921)

Freund (1990) comes to a similar conclusion in an article entitled 'The Expressive Body: a common ground for the sociology of the emotions and health and illness',

> To the extent to which this reconstruction and the stress of distressing experiences are chronic and encountered at junctures of biographical vulnerability, they may affect our health.
>
> (Freund 1990)

Karlsen and Nazroo (2002) challenge the notion that ethnic identity is related to health. They argue from the basis of their secondary analysis of the Fourth National Survey of Ethnic Minorities that while at first it does appear to be related to health status, when they carried out a multivariate factor analysis, it was experience of racism which was 'the only one that exhibited any relationship with health'. There are two points to note about this finding however: first, no Irish are identified as being in the large sample of ethnic minorities; second, it introduces the question of racism and whether the experiences of the Irish in England should be considered as racism.

The Report of the Commission for Racial Equality describes a wide range of discrimination against Irish people. The authors note that in their pilot survey,

25 per cent of those interviewed reported negative responses from police ranging from one case of serious assault to more commonplace verbal harassment... Discriminatory treatment at benefit offices was also described by 24 per cent of the sample.

(Hickman and Walter 1997: 235)

Although they recognise that the Irish were not then accepted as being a distinctive ethnic group, and that there was some disagreement about it amongst the Irish community, they feel confident in saying that ' The survey revealed a significant degree of anti-Irish racism...' (ibid: 237).

Whether they are right to define the discrimination which they and many other researchers including ourselves have found as racism, is still a matter for debate. Certainly the experience of difference is widespread, affecting men and women and people in all social classes; this 'felt' difference appears also to be institutionalised in that it is of long duration (Foster 1995), affects the quality of housing that Irish people are able to obtain (Harrison and Carr-Hill 1992; Cara 1994; Leonard 1999), and their experiences at benefit offices (Hickman and Walter, ibid). It may also be part of the 'institution-alised racism' as some of our respondents report and as noted by Hickman and Walter in their report for the CRE (ibid).

None of this makes the case for seeing the identity of the Irish in England as being essentially different. However, Brah (1996) makes a complex argu-ment to justify her position distinguishing essential differences from con-structed ones. She argues that identities are 'inscribed through experiences culturally constructed in social relations' but these identities are always in a state of flux although, in particular social and historically constructed con-texts they do gel around a core that is the residual one that is narratively carrying on the thread of their lives. This joining up of their experiences in England to the existing narrative of their lives is what is problematic for many Irish people, we suggest. Brah next introduces the concept of the collective identity

The process of signification whereby commonalities of experience around a specific axis of differentiation, say class, caste or religion, are invested with particular meaning.

(Brah 1996: 124)

She develops the argument further by saying that the emphasis put on one aspect of a person's identity, say their Irishness, will cause other more het-erogeneous aspects to partially dissolve. This process though is the result of historical and political discourses and the present context that Irish people in England inhabit and in that these can be subject to revision, it may not be appropriate to see the Irish experience as racism. Brah states that she sees racism as occurring between groups with 'fixed and immutable boundaries between groups signified as inherently different' and that

> power is performatively constituted in and through economic, political, and cultural practices. Subjectivities of both the dominant and dominated are produced in the interstices of these multiple, intersecting loci of power.
>
> (ibid: 125)

She then quotes from Stuart Hall (1992) who points to the way in which multiculturalist discourse has used the concept ethnicity to cover up the 'realities of racism and repression' before concluding, however, by saying that the concept of ethnicity may also be appropriated by those who use it to signify fixed differences between groups they see as inferior. Walter (2001) sees the English categorisation of Irish difference as clearly racist. She notes,

> The Irish have been represented as racially inferior since at least the twelfth century ... Thus the racialisation of the Irish is so ingrained in British culture as to be barely recognisable for what it is. Moreover there is now deep resistance among white British people to acknowledging it.
>
> (Walter 2001: 81)

Interestingly she argues that the position of the Irish in the United States is not the same as they are now constructed as 'white', illustrating the point that it is an historical and political process.

Whether the view the English take of Irish people is to see their differences as immutable and therefore racist remains an ongoing argument; whether the fact that it has been based on experience ongoing for more than two hundred years is the clinching fact remains a matter of fine judgement. What is clear is that their difference is experienced in a way which makes the development of identity precarious.

Conclusion

The main argument made in this chapter is that the poor health of the Irish in Britain may be partly explained by the problems they experience with identity. The difficulty of the Irish, as Bauman (2001) puts it, is not how to attain the identity of their choice but how to decide which identity to choose and have recognised by others; for the Irish as an emigrant group, some would say an exiled one, this is part of their daily experience as one of those interviewed eloquently said,

It's hard to know exactly what you want. It depends on how much you think about it … It depends on how you view yourself, whether you have succeeded in what you want over here, or whether you've failed and where you are going

(man in his 30s, interview 14)

Others made the same point less explicitly when they talked ruefully about making a visit home wearing their only suit with the only money they had in their pocket being last week's wages and being thought wealthy. Their identity problem was when they went back to the local environment of small-town-Ireland they did not fit in and nor did they when they were in the global environment of London where the daily hassle was to struggle to avoid being seen as simply the English 'other'. This 'felt' experience made it difficult to develop an authentic self and this experience it is argued has been to the detriment of both physical and mental health.

It might be said that they no longer experience the racism of the 'No Blacks No Irish' period of the 60s and 70s and that it is now 'trendy' to be Irish but the experience of those interviewed is powerful testimony to the fact that the recognition of difference is not easily erased and an authentic identity not easily achieved.

References

Antonosky A. (1963) 'Like Everyone Else, Only More So; identity, anxiety and the Jew' in A. Vidich and M. White (eds) *Identity and Anxiety*, USA Free Press.

Balarajan R. (1995) 'Ethnicity and Variations in the Nation's Health', *Health Trends*, 27, no. 4: 114–9.

Blumer H. (1969) 'Sociological Implications of the Thought of George Herbert Mead' in Herbert Blumer *Symbolic Interactionism*, London, University of California Press Ltd.

Bracken P., Greenslade L., Griffin B. and Smythe M. (1998) 'Mental Health and Ethnicity: an Irish Dimension', *British Journal of Psychiatry*, 172, 103–5.

Brah A. (1992) 'Difference, Diversity and Differentiation' in J. Donald and A. Rattansi (eds) *Race, Culture & Difference*, London, Sage.

Buckley M. (1997) 'Sitting on your Politics: the Irish among the British and the Women among the Irish' in Mac Laughlin (ed.) *Location and Dislocation in Contemporary Irish Society*, Cork, Cork University Press.

Chamberlin K. and Zika S. (1990) 'The minor events approach to stress: Support for the use of daily hassles', *British Journal of Psychology*, 81, 469–81.

Derrida J. (1978) *Writing and Difference*, Chicago, University of Chicago Press.

DeLongis A., Coyne J., Dakoff G., Folkman S. and Lazarus R. (1982) 'Relationship of daily hassles, uplifts, and major life events to health status', *Health Psychology* 1, (2) 119–36.

Economic and Social Research Institute of Ireland (1991) *Economic and Social Implications of Emigration*, National Economic and Social Council Report no. 90, Dublin, unpublished report.

Foster R.F. (1993) *Paddy and Mr. Punch*, London, Penguin Press.

Freund P. (1990) 'The expressive body : a common ground for the sociology of the emotions and health and illness, *Sociology of Health and Illness*, 12, 4.

Giddens A. (1991) *Modernity and Self-Identity*, Cambridge, Polity Press.

Habermas J. (1987) *The theory of Communicative Action*, vol. 2, Cambridge, Polity Press.

Hall S. (1994) 'The question of cultural identity' in *Cultural Theory*, Cambridge, Polity Press.

Harrison L. and Carr-Hill R. (1992) *Alcohol and Disadvantage Amongst the Irish in England*, Hull, Department of Social Policy, University of Hull.

Hickman M. and Walter B. (1997) *Discrimination and the Irish Community in Britain*, London, Commission for Racial Equality.

Kaplan H. (1991) 'Social psychology of the immune system: a conceptual framework and review of the literature, *Social Science and Medicine*, 33, 8: 909–23.

Kelleher D. and Hillier S. (1996) 'The Health of the Irish in England' in D. Kelleher and S. Hillier *Researching Cultural Differences in Health*, London, Routledge .

Leavey G. (1999) 'Suicide and Irish Migrants in Britain: identity and integration', *International Review of Psychiatry*, 11, 168–72.

MacLauglin (ed) (2000) 'Changing attitudes to "new wave" emigration? Structuralism versus voluntarism in the study of Irish emigration' in *The Irish Diaspora*, Harlow, Pearson Education Ltd.

Mead G.H. (1934) *Mind, Self, and Society* in C. H. Morris (ed.), Chicago, University of Chicago Press.

Miller K. (1990) 'Emigration, capitalism and ideology in post famine Ireland' in R. Kearney (ed) *Migrations: The Irish at Home and Abroad*, Dublin, Wolfhound Press.

O'Connell M. (2001) *Changed Utterly*, Dublin, The Liffey Press.

Rutherford J. (1990) 'A place called home: identity and the cultural politics of Difference' in J. Rutherford (ed.) *Identity*, London, Lawrence and Wishart.

Steptoe A. (1991) 'The links between stress and illness', *Journal of Psychosomatic Research*, 35, 6. 633–44.

Tilki M. (1996) 'The Health of the Irish in Britain', *FIS Bulletin*, May.

Walter B. (2001) *Outsiders Inside*, London, Routledge.

Winston N. (2000) *Between Two Places*, Dublin, Irish National Committee of the European Cultural Foundation.

6

Sport, health and identity: social and cultural change in disorganised capitalism

Graham Scambler, Steffan Ohlsson and Konstadina Griva

The positive association between sport and health has a long pedigree in Britain and elsewhere. What have varied are the interpretations of this association and the sets of social relations in which sport, health and the interpretations themselves have been embedded. In the opening section of this chapter we offer an outline account of the transition from what, following numerous precedents, we shall term 'organised' to 'disorganised capitalism'. In the course of this account the renewed salience and defining properties of the notion of 'identity' will be touched on. The second section considers in more detail the linkages between sport, health and identity in disorganised capitalism, that is, in the period from the mid-1970s to the present. A general typology of exercise, sport and health risk is advanced. The focus of the third and final section is on professional sport in general and rugby union in particular. Our reflections on the changed parameters of professional rugby allow further refinements of the case we make for a re-theorisation of the association between sport and health in contemporary Britain.

From organised to disorganised capitalism

It may be helpful to start with broad characterisations of organised and disorganised capitalism. Fortunately not all of the changes that have marked this transition are pertinent to the argument of this chapter, so we can be selective. It should be noted too that for all the multiplicity of changes that have occurred over the last generation, *much has remained unchanged*: it has become all too customary to lose a sense of continuity in fashionable pursuit of discontinuity. The discontinuities/continuities we wish to emphasise can be epitomised in a family of six themes that cut across distinctions made elsewhere between the 'material', the 'cultural-aesthetic', the 'rational' and the 'methodological' (Scambler 2002). They focus on:

1. aspects of a conspicuous economic and cultural globalisation (or, more precisely, 'glocalisation');

2. the renewed salience of relations of class and their partial usurpation of relations of command;
3. the persistence of class habitus despite the diminishing relevance of ('objective') class for ('subjective') identity formation;
4. the enhanced pace of individualisation;
5. the general post-modernisation of culture; and
6. the politically honed filtering of power in terms of Foucauldian 'technologies of the self' and 'governmentality'.

We shall briefly consider each theme in turn.

Globalising tendencies

The past is characterised by waves of diverse forms of globalisation, and considerable caution is required in any assessment of its nature and extent in disorganised capitalism. No single member of Held and colleagues' (1999) triad of ideal types – the 'hyperglobalist', the 'sceptic' or the 'transformationalist' – can yet be said to have had the final say. There is clear evidence, however, of tendencies central to this chapter. Transnational corporations have undoubtedly achieved pre-eminence in world output, trade, investment and technology transfer. Even more dramatically, the extensity, intensity, velocity and impact of global financial flows – that is, relative to global or national output – are unprecedented: whereas, historically, trading in foreign exchange was a product of transnational trade, trade at the start of the millennium accounted for a mere 2 per cent of global currency movements. Largely liquid, global financial flows are attracted by short- term speculative gains and carry a potential to salvage or savage national economies. Some, like Sklair (2000), contend that there now exists a transnational capitalist class, while others, like Scott (1997), regard this as a somewhat premature if understandable judgement.

These economic aspects of globalisation have been accompanied by, and we wish to add are in part responsible for, cultural shifts. But there is more to these than a putative Americanisation or 'MacDonaldisation' of world culture. A prerequisite for globalisation, Giddens (1990) insists, has been the distanciation or separation of time and space, which has allowed for the 'disembedding' or 'lifting out' of social relations from their local contexts, principally through expert systems, like repositories of technical knowledge, and symbolic tokens, like money. Accompanying the advent of the truly global has been a reinvigoration of the local, hence Robertson's (1992) coinage of the term 'glocalisation'. The local, however, is no longer *merely local*, but rather can be readily accessed and marketed, globally.

Changing relations of class and command

Much has been written of the decline of the nation state occasioned by the globalising tendencies of the capitalist economy, although analysts like Weiss (1999) have rightly stressed that this decline is more marked in some nation states than in others, and that it is in any case a matter always of degree. Another way of framing the changing relationship between the strongly globalised capitalist-executives heading transnational corporations and the weakly globalised power-elites governing nation states is in terms of relations of class and command. Bluntly expressed, relations of command have ceded ground to relations of class (Scambler 2002). Far from relations of class diminishing in significance in disorganised capitalism (as has often been claimed, some even announcing the 'death of class') (Pakulski and Waters 1996), they have become reinvigorated, and in the process first, constraints on capitalist-executives' pursuits of profit have been progressively removed, and second, the capacities and will of power-elites to respond to the working class, let alone the 'new poor', have been progressively curtailed.

Class habitus and identity formation

One of the most attractive properties of Bourdieu's (1977) concept of 'habitus' is its potential to help us understand the growing disjunction in disorganised capitalism between the *objective* relations of class addressed in theme (2) and *subjective* relations of class. Habitus refers to a set of 'lasting, transposable dispositions' generated by objective relations of class but not necessarily recognised in terms of (subjective relations of) class by those involved. While objective relations of class have 'become reinvigorated', there is no doubt that subjective relations of class, in this sense, have become far less pertinent than they were under either liberal or organised capitalism. One symptom of this is the diminished role people's sense of class membership plays in their perceptions of who they are and aspire to be. Note that this is not at all to say that objective relations of class have ceased to 'inform' either such interrogations of self or the answers arrived at.

Not only has people's sense of class membership become a less important ingredient in their self-definitions, identity formation has itself assumed a new significance in disorganised capitalism. As Bendle (2002: 1) puts it, the acquisition and maintenance of identity has become 'vital *and* problematic', although as yet these processes remain 'under-theorised'. He suggests the under-theorisation has occurred due to an imperative under globalisation to:

> theorize people as possessing identities that are extremely adaptive to social change. As a result, there is an inherent contradiction between a

valuing of identity as something so fundamental that it is crucial to personal well-being and collective action, and a theorization of 'identity' that sees it as something constructed, fluid, multiple, impermanent and fragmentary. The contemporary crisis of identity thus expresses itself as both a crisis of society, and a crisis of theory. The crisis of identity involves a crisis of 'identity'.

(Bendle 2002: 1–2).

We shall have more to say about both identity and 'identity' later.

Individualisation

In reviewing class and stratification in disorganised capitalism, Scott (2002) espouses the line on objective/subjective class relations expressed above. He goes on to argue, citing Beck (1992), that the diminution of class conscious-ness and 'weakening of class imagery' reflects growing processes of indi-vidualisation:

under the conditions of a radicalized or reflexive modernity, social identities relate much more to lifestyle differences in consumption, to differences in gender, sexuality and ethnicity, and to attempts to under-stand and control the risks and hazards generated by contemporary modernization'.

(Scott 2002: 33).

In the context of the 'new individualisation', class is but one source of identity among others.

However paradoxical it might appear, our contention is that the resur-gence of objective class relations in global or disorganised capitalism, not least *vis-à-vis* command relations, has been causally influential in both the new individualisation and the closely related, if derivative, foregrounding and splintering of identity formation. What is often presented as a displace-ment within the economic sector of productivism by consumerism since the mid-1970s, we see primarily as a shift at the cultural or ideological level. The post-modernisation of contemporary culture might reasonably be seen as the advent of a new 'culture-ideology of consumerism' (Sklair 2000), that is, as a further step towards the logical endpoint of the capitalist project, the 'commodification of everything' (Wallerstein 1998). To claim as much is not to strip culture of all its autonomy, but rather to affirm what has been termed the 'principle of compatibility': cultural innovation might take many and unpredictable forms, but, *ceteris paribus*, it is unlikely to take forms that are incompatible with the prevailing logics of the regime of capital accumulation and its mode of regulation (Scambler 2002: 66).

The post-modern culture

The designation of the culture of disorganised capitalism, or high or late modernity, as post-modern must be distinguished from any assertion of a transition to a novel social formation, or post-modernity. We have suggested that contemporary culture features a push towards individualisation and, to recall Bendle, a crisis of identity and 'identity'; and that, however else this might be interpreted, it is part and parcel of a culture-ideology of consumerism. But what, for the purposes at hand, are the key characteristics of what it is reasonable to call our post-modern culture? Vincent (2003: 110), in his study of old age, lists the following features:

- instability, insecurity, flexibility, rapid change, the breakdown of old certainties and social conditions without overarching values or fundamental principles;
- reflexivity, self-awareness, an ability to understand, control and manipulate ourselves and others in unprecedented ways;
- institutional arrangements which reflect these features, including consumerism, fluid family structures, temporary short-term contracts of employment, volatile global markets and identity politics;
- cultural manifestations of these features giving dominance to display, irony, multiple ambiguous meanings and appearance rather than essence.

Two characteristics warrant special emphasis in the context of this chapter. First, post-modern culture is generally and understandably associated with the loss of face and credibility of what Lyotard (1984) terms the 'metanarratives', or arch-theories, of post-Enlightenment capitalism/modernity, ranging from free-market liberalism to revolutionary Marxism. These *grand* narratives have been succeeded, Lyotard informs us, by a diverse and 'liberating' mosaic of equally credible/incredible *petit* narratives. One of us has taken note of this phenomenon, but argued that far from being liberating it represents (self-refuting) relativism in new clothing and, for all that it may appear 'disinhibiting', is ultimately neo-conservative (Scambler 1996; 2002). The second characteristic is our enhanced capacity for self-turnover (Scambler 2001). Amongst other things, petit narratives afford a multiplicity of equally credible/incredible and largely commodified resources for identity formation. It is easier in our post-modern culture not only to 'present' but to 'be' different by context and audience. It is now feasible not only to hold to positions that would formerly have been deemed contradictory but to construct and manage a repertoire of transposable identities.

Technologies of the self and governmentality

One of the virtues of Foucault's later work was his subtle appreciation of the multifarious ways in which power is routinely enacted beyond witting individual or collective acts of domination. This enactment is epitomised in his concept of 'technologies of the self'. Progressively from the late eighteenth century, Foucault (1980) contends, individuals have internalised pervasive, humanist discourses of, for example, healthy regimes to the extent that they have now come to retain under continuous surveillance and to 'police' their own behaviours. Thus medicine's contribution to 'social control' no longer takes the form of exclusion or repression, but rather of inclusion and normalisation. Technologies of the self are allied to what Foucault (1979) terms 'governmentality'. This refers to the 'conduct of conduct' or the 'government of government'. The external threat of coercion, in short, has given way to internal mechanisms of self-monitoring. In a sense we govern ourselves. Foucault's insights are shrewd and important, but they are too dismissive of domination. Power can exist without domination, but it continues also to be exercised through the latter. In our view, in the reflexive era of disorganised capitalism, this 'new' or Foucauldian form of power has been calculatingly honed as political technique and in part integrated into the command relations of the state. Moreover, command relations have become more responsive to class relations.

There is, of course, a great deal more that might profitably be said about Britain in the new millennium than is contained or even hinted at in the above six themes. But they provide a theoretical backcloth to the more specific focus on sport and health that follows and inform the analysis with which the chapter concludes.

Exercise, sport and health

The notion that sport, health and well-being are positively associated has long had currency and continues to do so independently of the transition from organised to disorganised capitalism:

> in developing and developed societies, in capitalist and communist societies and in democratic and totalitarian societies, there is a broad consensus that 'sport is good for you'
>
> (Waddington 2000: 408).

But the proposition that sport is good for you is at best simplistic and at worst obfuscatory. Setting aside for the moment the ideological baggage this proposition has almost always concealed, sport, to paraphrase Wittgenstein (1958), conjures up activities with no discernible core properties in common but rather with 'family resemblances'. Some sporting activities may be conducive to health and well-being, others not; and it is likely often to be a matter of degree. An expedient point of departure for us, therefore, is to offer a summary statement on the now extensive (neo-)positivist literature on linkages between sport and health.

Such a summary might sensibly begin by distinguishing between sport and *exercise*, since it is the latter that features in most (neo-)positivist studies. And these studies point with unusual consistency to the conclusion that 'moderate, rhythmic and regular exercise has a significant and beneficial impact on health' (Waddington 2000: 411). A report by the Royal College of Physicians (1991: 28) concludes that

> there is substantial evidence that regular aerobic exercise such as walking, jogging, dancing or swimming is beneficial to general physical and psychological health'.

It continues:

> regular exercise appears to be particularly effective in the prevention of coronary disease and osteoporosis and of some value in the management of obesity and diabetes.

Analyses of insurance statistics suggest that regular exercise is a significant non-pharmacological method of lowering blood pressure (and men with low blood pressure can expect to live 15 years longer than men with only moderately high blood pressure) (BMA 1992). One American study reports that mortality rates among men whose work or leisure involves regular exercise are between one-third and one-half lower than those among men whose lives are more sedentary (Paffenbarger *et al.* 1986). Reviewing the international evidence, Smith and Jacobson (1988) conclude that the protective effects of regular exercise

1. persist at all ages, even after other 'risk factors' like smoking and weight are taken into account;
2. can be produced relatively quickly – in a three-month period – in both men and women of all ages, although they are maintained only while the activity is maintained; and
3. are most apparent in those who are least active, especially older people or those with chronic conditions.

Even allowing for the worrying (neo-)positivist propensity to impute causality on the basis of statistical association, reflecting an abiding commitment to the flawed Humean regularity theory of causation (Scambler 2002), there is enough 'evidence' to posit beneficial effects for health from moderate, rhythmic and regular exercise, that is, exercise ranging from 'brisk walking, running or swimming for 20–30 minutes about three times each week' (Smith and Jacobson 1988: 126), to 'energetic getting about' or the regular climbing of stairs for older people (Morris *et al.* 1980).

Participation in these forms of exercise also seems to bring benefits in terms of psychological health and well-being (Eastbrooks *et al.* 2003). Large-scale epidemiological studies suggest that exercise is associated with positive affect and mood, and conversely, that physical inactivity is associated with more negative emotions (see Biddle *et al.* 2000). In terms of mental health, it appears that exercise can reduce anxiety to some degree and clinical depression rather more (Lawlor and Hopker 2001). The mechanisms responsible for these effects are not well understood, although a number have been hypothesised, ranging from positive effects on self-efficacy and self-esteem to increased levels of serontin. Evidence-based guidelines from health authorities suggest that whether a person is exercising on his or her own or in a group, it is a focus on self-development, effort and mastery of tasks that most impact on mood and psychological well-being (Grant 2000). This 'task orientation' is compared favourably to 'ego orientation', where exercisers strive to be better than others and where a competitive ethos prevails. As we shall see, research on professional and/or elite sport indicates that engagement in the competitive sports arena can be linked to adverse psychological outcomes.

Exercise and sport may be 'overlapping activities' but there are nevertheless important differences between them (Waddington 2000). It is, for example, revealing that a study of competitive athletes in New Zealand conducted by Sullivan and colleagues (1994) found positive associations between 'intense exercise' and competition-induced anxiety, stitches, lightheadedness, muscle cramps, wheezing, chest pressure, spots before the eyes, retching and incontinence of urine and stool; negative associations were reported with fewer symptoms, amongst them headaches, abdominal bloating, sneezing and depression. Sport for most sociologists is inherently competitive. Waddington (2000: 413) notes, in general, that non-competitive exercise and competitive sport involve different sets of social relations; and, in particular, that the former is more likely than the latter to involve rhythmic movements and to be under the control of the individual participant. Sport is the more complex activity (see Elias and Dunning 1986). Given the 'game pattern' of most sports, the individual participant has no choice but to cede control over his or her own movements and the pace and intensity at which he or she is able to play. Movement easily becomes the antithesis of rhythmic and bursts of anaerobic activity become paradigmatic (Waddington 2000).

The degree to and intensity with which sport has been competitive has varied historically (Scambler forthcoming), but it is part of the contention of this chapter that sport's 'professionalisation' in disorganised capitalism has considerably augmented what has been identified as a post-war trend. 'To succeed in modern sport', Donohoe and Johnson (1986: 93) maintain:

> athletes are forced to train longer, harder, and earlier in life. They may be rewarded by faster times, better performances and increased fitness, but there is a price to pay for such intense training.

One such price is a threat to health. Unsurprisingly this threat is most apparent at the elite level.

Waddington quotes from a number of accounts from elite athletes indicating health threats beyond mere training intensity. The Soviet gymnast Olga Korbut, gold-medal winner in the Munich Olympic Games, reported on a tour of Germany following the Games:

> during that tour of Germany, the lumbago in my back began to hurt more and more. The novocaine injections took away the pain for a while, but I needed time to rest and heal. By the end of the tour, I walked as though I had a stake in my spine . . .

She continued:

> my strongest memory of that entire period are fatigue, pain, and the empty feeling of being a fly whose blood has been sucked out by a predatory spider.
>
> (Korbut 1992: 81–2).

Waddington also reproduces a telling extract from a pre-match team talk given by coach John Monie to the Wigan rugby league players:

> There's just one more thing I want to enforce. It doesn't matter what's wrong with you when you're injured, I want you on your feet and in the defensive line . . . I don't care if the physio's out there and he wants to examine you and all that stuff. That's not important. What's important is . . . you've got twelve team-mates tackling their guts out, defending like anything inside the 22 and we've got the physio telling a guy to see if he can straighten his knee out. I don't care what's wrong with you . . . if the opposition's got the ball, I want you on your feet and in the defensive line . . . There are no exceptions to that rule. So from now on, the only reason you stay down hurt and get attention from the sideline is because there's a break in play or you're unconscious – no other reasons will be accepted.
>
> (Hanson 1991: 77).

Young (1993) has recorded this same mind-set amongst coaches in the American NFL ('you play unless the bone sticks through the meat'). Not infrequently, Hanson found, Wigan players only started matches courtesy of pain-killing injections. Former England soccer captain Gary Lineker also resented the routine use of pain-killing injections, commenting on his retirement (occasioned by a chronic foot injury):

> it is as if a huge weight has been lifted from me. I no longer have to worry whether I'll be fit enough to get through a match and I will no longer have to suffer the dizzy spells and stomach complaints that come with a dependency on anti-inflammatory drugs.
>
> (quoted in Waddington 2000: 416).

Overuse injury is extremely common in elite sport. Young and colleagues (1994: 190) from the USA once more:

> overt and covert pressures are brought to bear on injured athletes to coerce them to return to action. These may include certain 'degradation ceremonies' ... such as meal areas, constant questioning from coaches, being ostracised at team functions, or other special treatment that clearly identifies the injured athlete as separate.

One study of 123 Danish soccer players found that 37 per cent of injuries were overuse injuries (Lynch and Carcasona 1994). According to FIFA's report on soccer's World Cup in 1994, 12 per cent of all treatments of players were for chronic injuries or ailments that predated the Finals in the USA (Nepfer 1994). But, as Waddington points out, such injuries are not, or are no longer, confined to elite competitors. A survey conducted in England and Wales for the Sports Council discovered that one-third of all injuries resulting from participation in sport/exercise were recurrent injuries. Extrapolating from these data, the Sports Council estimated there are 10.4 million incidents per annum leading to recurrent injuries (that is, in addition to 19.3 million resulting in new injuries) (Sports Council 1991: 25).

The Sports Council also distinguished different sports by risk of injury. Top of the list was rugby, with an injury rate of 59 per 100 participants per four weeks. Second in dangerousness was soccer (39), followed by martial arts (36), hockey (25) and cricket (20). Rugby also headed the list of high-risk sports in a New Zealand study (Hume and Marshall 1994). Clearly a number of distinctions are relevant to the differential risk of injury. The distinction between exercise and sport remains basic and has already been adumbrated. To this might be added others, for example between (professional) elite and (amateur) mass sport, and between contact and non-contact sports. Of elite contact sports in the USA, Young (1993: 373) bluntly and unambiguously writes:

by any measure, professional sport is a violent and hazardous work-
place, replete with its own unique forms of 'industrial disease'. No other
milieu, including the risky and labour-intensive settings of miners, oil
drillers, or construction site workers, can compare with the routine
injuries of team sports such as football, ice-hockey, soccer, rugby and
the like.

There are sufficient empirical data to justify a rudimentary typology of
exercise/sports – and, for the purposes of this chapter, their associated
identity tags (plus exemplars) – ranked by increasing health threat. Such a
typology might reasonably comprise the following:

1. Exercise   *(the exerciser*: e.g. jogging)
2. Non-competitive sport   *(the enthusiast*: e.g. orienteering)
3. Non-contact competitive sport   *(the competitor*: e.g. tennis)
4. Contact competitive sport   *(the contester*: e.g. rugby)
5. Combat competitive sport   *(the gladiator*: e.g. boxing)
6. Dangerous sport   *(the gambler*: e.g. mountaineering)

Only 1) might be described as generally health bestowing, although 2) to 6)
will intermittently accommodate elements of 1) (not least in elements of
training). There is of course nothing sacrosanct about the particular identity
labels attached to each of these pursuits. Moreover, many individuals would
lay legitimate claim to proprietorship of more than one label, and many
activities can be assigned to more than one category (swimming, for example, can be a form of exercise, a non-competitive sport and a non-contact
competitive sport). The examples given should be regarded as paradigmatic,
serving merely to empirically 'anchor' the categories. The typology serves
a heuristic purpose here.

   The centrality of lifestyle and consumer choice – extending to exercise and
sport – to people's identities is a singular feature of disorganised capitalism.
As such, it warrants a further brief comment before we turn in more detail to
the contesters of elite professional rugby union. Consider the identity of the
exerciser. This is typically now about far more than health enhancement. To
many exercisers, no less important than the health return on exercise are
other altogether more aesthetic aspects of 'body maintenance'. In our post-
modern culture or, more sociologically and more in line with the argument
of this chapter, in accordance with the culture-ideology of consumerism, the
body has become a site of pleasure and a representation of happiness and
success. Nettleton's (1995) suggestion that nowadays 'to look good is to *feel*
good' might be extended to read: 'to look good is to look healthy is to *feel*
good is to *feel* healthy'. Common to the media treatment of body maintenance and to health promotion programmes is the encouragement of self-
surveillance of bodily appearance and health, with the incentive of lifestyle

benefits also very much to the fore. According to Featherstone (1991), there has been a 'transvaluation' of activities such as jogging, which have been freshly evaluated in light of their putative health benefits. The most conspicuous outcome of the resultant commodification of healthy lifestyles is the 'fitness industry': its products ranging widely and loosely from exercise machines to stylish and branded clothing.

A study that illustrates in an interesting but paradoxical way the post-modern notion that 'to look good is to look healthy is to *feel* good is to *feel* healthy' is Monaghan's (2001) on bodybuilding. In one of several reports of his ethnographic study of bodybuilding subculture, the author sets about making good medical sociology's neglect of health and well-being (Monaghan 2001a). For those embroiled in 'the positive moment' of body-building, he avers, this kind of activity is seen as beneficial to mental, physical and/or social health. In fact, the gym culture of which such individuals are part largely consists of Foucauldian 'technologies of the self' which are affected by 'normalized subjects in pursuit of self-improvement, happiness and healthiness' (Monaghan 2001a: 332). A question Monaghan poses is: why are bodybuilders willing to engage in potentially health-damaging practices, even extending to illicit drug use, to secure 'strong, fit and healthy-looking bodies'? Although bodybuilding *can* be addictive, he maintains that it is not satisfactory either to pathologise the commitment to bodybuilding and steroid use in terms of personal or gender inadequacy (see, for example, Klein 1993; 1995), or to medicalise this same commitment as the product of reverse anorexia or muscle dysmorphia (see Pope *et al.* 2000). 'More positive' readings than these are possible (Monaghan 2002).

Monaghan (2001a: 334) argues that there is a degree of overlap between bodybuilders and our category of exercisers: namely, they share an attempt to 'embody and display a sense of empowerment and self-mastery'. However, for all that bodybuilding has been described as health-enhancing, 'many participants know lifting weights is primarily an anaerobic as opposed to aerobic activity'. Bodybuilding requires relatively little cardio-vascular fitness which health promoters consider so important for physical health. Indeed, the primary goal of bodybuilding is 'the look' – to change one's body appearance so that it more or less approximates idealised images of health, youth, fitness and beauty (Featherstone, 1991) rather than to confer any direct benefit in internal physiological functioning (Monaghan 2001a: 337). It is the health of the 'outer body' that is important. As far as bodybuilders are concerned, then, the embodied pleasures and perceived psychosocial benefits of anaerobic exercise, combined with the 'post-modern imagery of muscle', are typically of high significance in sustaining the 'ongoing consumption of (risky) bodybuilding technologies' (Monaghan 2001a: 335).

The following sequence of quotations from Monaghan's respondents is revealing of his underlying themes:

... the thing about bodybuilding is that you can look fit even if you're not. That's the thing about bodybuilders. They look tremendous.

It's all to do with looks, and I would rather look good on the outside. That's what bodybuilding is. It's not for fitness reasons'.

You look fit. People always remark how fit I look even when I'm tired. They always say 'you look really fit and healthy' and they used to say that to me when I was dieting (for a bodybuilding competition): 'you look great, your eyes are shining, your skin is clear'.

They're both important, but looking healthy I think is the key rather than being healthy ... But one complements the other. Because if you look healthy you're going to feel healthy. You're going to feel healthier anyway aren't you?'

... I think if you appear with a good physique and look after your physique and get back into training, you look good, feel good and I think that wards off quite a few problems. But it is more important to look good, feel good, because that relates then doesn't it?

I would always like to think that people always come up to me and say: 'well, fair play, you look fit sort of thing'. And going to my doctor, he says: 'well you're fit' ... But you know, like I say, it (looking and being healthy) is combined. It's a mixture of the two.

When I go down to the gym, I go there with a goal in mind, and when I come out of there I nearly always feel that I've had a brilliant workout. 'God, that was brilliant!' I feel powerful, I feel strong, I feel energetic. It's just a nice feeling. But I don't know any other sport that you can get that sort of rush every workout almost.

Training, diet and controlled steroid use enable bodybuilders to look and feel younger, fitter and healthier for longer. And the 'steroid pump', discussed by Monaghan under the rubric of the 'erotics of the gym', can give bodybuilders a real high. Arnold Schwarzenegger elaborates:

The greatest feeling you can get in the gym or the most satisfying feeling you can get in the gym is *the Pump*. Let's say you train your biceps: blood is rushing into your muscles and that's what we call 'the Pump'. Your muscles get a really *tight feeling*, like your skin is going to explode any minute. You know it's really tight like somebody is blowing air into your muscles. It just blows up and it feels different, it feels fantastic. It's as satisfying to me as *coming* is, you know, as having sex with a woman and coming. *So you can believe how much I am in heaven*!

(see Wacquant 1995: 176).

Monaghan (2001a: 351) readily admits that bodybuilding may entail physically detrimental practices, including illicit drug use, especially amongst 'hard-core' physique competitors. But he also finds in the activities of bodybuilders a 'situated rationality' articulated through the pleasures implicit in their ascetic lifestyle:

> their sense of physical and emotional wellbeing derived from achieving 'the look', their learnt capacity to enjoy intense physical exercise and the perceived benefits for everyday pragmatic embodiment.

The relevance of Monaghan's intriguing analysis here is that it illustrates just what lies the other side of health-bestowing exercise in our post-modern culture. Healthy exercise is often on the cusp of transmutation through a pursuit of identity for self and others that provides a key focus and rationale for a hugely profitable fitness industry. Again, much of what passes for post-modern freedom to forge novel and appealing personal identities in fact reflects the hypercommodification characteristic of global or disorganised capitalism. Paradoxically, the price paid for looking and feeling good, and therefore looking and feeling healthy, a potent and positive statement of contemporary youthful identity, may be health risk or even declining health status. This dynamic around sport/exercise, health and identity has become pivotal, and it has its impact on each category in our typology, not least on the contesters of contact competitive sport, to which – in the form of professional rugby union – we now turn in more detail.

The contesters of professional rugby

Rugby union was officially declared an open game as late as 1995, but any sense that this marked its unambiguous transition from an amateur to a professional sport requires qualification. It is true that rugby was from the outset characterised by the amateur ethos of the English public school; and that in its earliest days 'professionalism' – namely, taking games seriously enough to plan and prepare to win them – was deemed 'tantamount to transforming it into work, and, hence, to destroy its essence' (Dunning and Sheard 1979: 148). But by the 1880s, rugby had already become a spectator sport, with clubs charging their supporters entry fees. This had a twofold effect: clubs wanted teams to improve on performance to notch up victories to attract support, and paying spectators wanted to see good games. Rugby rapidly became 'professional' according to the definition of the Victorian era. Teams strove to win and preparation was a necessary condition for success.

New cup and league competitions exacerbated this process, with players being 'subsidised' or allotted generous travelling expenses to play. Eventually, in 1895, the game was fractured, bifurcated into its two forms: (southern, middle-class amateur) union, emphasising unpaid leisure, and (northern, working-class professional) league, emphasising paid work (Dunning and Sheard, 1979). This bifurcation stuck for a century, although by the time of the transition from organised to disorganised capitalism in the early 1970s little was left of amateurism in either its Victorian or more modern senses, at least amongst the leading national or club teams.

We have already noted the health and injury hazards that accompany playing rugby, where a high degree of physical contact is of the essence of the game, risks compounded in the newly commercialised game emergent in the 1960s and 1970s and further accelerated in the years since 1995. British journalist, Paul Rees (2003), refers to an Australian study of elite players showing that while in the year before the game went open there were 47 injuries per 1000 player-hours, that figure increased by nearly 50 per cent to 69 injuries per 1000 player-hours, with 143 injuries recorded from 91 matches, in the following year. The fly-half was the most injured back and the lock the most injured forward. Rees (2003) quotes Bristol coach Peter Thorburn:

> there is a conflict in the sport between the commercial and the playing sides. Clubs want to generate more money to balance the books but the risk is that too much is asked of the players. It is not just about matches, though I think there are too many: we have contact training twice a week, and even though players wear protective suits there is the risk of injury ... The trouble with the British season is that there is little let-up in it. Once you start in September, you are involved in a non-stop process of build-up and playing. There is little room for recovery. Staleness and boredom creep in and injuries pile up. The busiest members of a club's management are the physio and the masseur ... Players may be well paid but that does not mean we have bought their hearts and bodies. There is a danger we will turn them into a scrapheap ...

This notion of professional clubs 'getting their monies worth' features in an unpublished account by one of the authors of this chapter, from which the player statements below are taken (Ohlsson 2001). Focusing on senior Premiership Division RFCs in Wales, Ohlsson distinguishes six phases in the professional rugby player's career: the development phase, the professional phase, the establishment phase, the maximisation phase, the pre-retirement phase and the retirement phase. The development phase sees players through school and youth squad rugby, ending when the chosen few sign at 18 years or later for a senior club. Signing a contract with a senior club, not permissible before 18, signifies entry to the professional phase, although club scouts may be expected to pick out and approach outstanding talent from youth squads earlier than this. The establishment phase marks players securing their positions in the senior club. The maximisation phase finds players fulfilling their individual potentials, in terms of their playing abilities, ambitions (for example, for international honours), status in the community, and income. By the time of the pre-retirement phase, players are anticipating their post-rugby careers, often becoming more instrumental in the process. Finally, in the retirement phase, players adjust, or do not adjust, to their futures off the pitch.

Ohlsson makes the point that injury can inhibit, even terminate, accomplishment and ambition as early as the development phase, and at any time during the professional, establishment, maximisation and pre-retirement phases. Talent at this level is no longer enough: players have to be bigger, stronger, quicker and to show greater endurance than in previous eras. Ohlsson reports two ways in which players might stay ahead of their competitors: physical and psychological preparation. The former refers to achieving higher levels of strength, power, speed, skill and fitness. This extends beyond training regimes to encompass a range of lifestyle factors. Diet, for example, has become vital:

> I've tried different proteins, shakes, energy drinks, things like that, but you sit with a dietitian and have a chat ... More than anything the only performance enhancer at the moment is plenty of water. As simple as it sounds, that is one of the best lessons I ever learnt.

As one player put it:

> basically your whole lifestyle is geared around performing on a Saturday.

Not merely diet but alcohol intake, and the socialising rituals in which this is often embedded, have to be monitored and curtailed. Even players in the retirement phase can feel too guilty to relax on a Saturday. As one former Welsh and Lions captain put it:

> I feel now when I cover a game or go and watch my old club I can't go and have a pint after the game. I never go for a pint because I don't feel I've earned it. I have to go and run and train, and get a sweat on – you know, it's that satisfaction of doing it.

A number of contemporary professional players take 'legal' performance enhancing supplements such as protein and weight-gain powders and it would be disingenuous to deny that some also take 'illegal' performance enhancing anabolic steroids.

Psychological preparation too is becoming integral to commercial rugby union, not least because physical preparation can reach such a pitch that players 'cancel each other out'. Sports psychologists have become commonplace in Welsh rugby union since the late 1980s. As one player expressed it:

> A lot of work goes into making everyone mentally tip-top. Everyone's got to be on, well, the edge really, and I think it's preparing yourself for the week with your food intake, your fluid intake, and obviously mental preparation as well ... certain things like visualisation now, there's a lot of it coming into rugby. These psychologists are poking into every kind of club to try to get the best performance, and I think it's more now preparation off the field, mentally ... than actually doing it, physically, on a training field.

Players have to be 'mentally on the ball' for each match; but they also, as Peter Thorburn, emphasises above, have to survive arduous and more and more protracted seasons without succumbing to mental fatigue, even burnout. One Welsh international and British Lion catches the tension well:

> I get over it by escaping, by going away and spending quality time with the family. By doing more relaxing things, getting away more and doing a bit more of the cinema. Maybe not going out for a Saturday night out after a game, you know. Don't go out on a Saturday night, don't drink, and you don't feel bad on a Sunday ... Chill and really have quality time with your family and friends and girlfriend, or whatever. Have a bit of quality time with yourself ... For all the intents and purposes, do nothing. Because, you know, I was mentally tired coming into the season, and I was a little disillusioned because I had some people from the A team saying this, and I had Graham Henry contradicting them and saying he wanted this from me; and I had to turn to my club coach, you know, just to get back to my game and to get focused. For the last six games of the season it was hard. I think sometimes the body gets a battering, and I think with my club we're pretty good because we've got 'X', who is a great guy, he's intelligent and he listens to players. I think the one thing is mentally, you know, you mentally being on the ball.

Howe (2001) offers a more focused and extremely insightful ethnographic account of pain and injury amongst rugby players in his study of a single Welsh club, Pontypridd RFC. Having duly registered the high risks, he acknowledges that the elimination of injury to players has become a 'paramount performative, and therefore financial, concern'. One focus of research interest for Howe is the expectation and accommodation of injury as one of a complex of factors that comprise the habitus of a professional rugby club. Bourdieu's (1977) concept of habitus was briefly encountered earlier in this chapter in relation to class. Bourdieu (1988; 1993) was of course himself interested in sport. Howe (2001: 292) adopts his notion to refer to the 'habitual, embodied practices that collectively comprise and define a culture', in this instance that of Pontypridd RFC. Rugby clubs, like professional soccer clubs, might be expected to be protective and encompassing, to afford opportunities for the addictive excitement and intensity of playing, and a subculture of camaraderie (Gearing 1999).

At the heart of the habitus of Pontypridd RFC is a determination to succeed on behalf of the club (Howe 1997). No longer a 'community cooperative', processes of commercialisation, or commodification, have transformed the club into a potentially lucrative business enterprise, with economic gain becoming more important than 'championing community identity' (Howe 1999). This commodification of the sport has been paralleled by the players' professionalisation. Professionalisation brought in its wake increasing, and increasingly intense, training schedules and associated rates of injury. In this way, Howe argues, the changing habitus of the club has had a direct effect on players' personal and social experience of pain and injury. Such is the salience of body capital for the elite athlete that what would pass as acute pain for an amateur or non-sportsperson becomes chronic pain for a professional obliged to forego training.

Howe found that in general if a player, say, broke his arm, the pain was obvious but then 'disappeared' in the sense that no reference was subsequently made to it, while if an injury was 'playable' then the player would let it be known that he was in pain. This latter strategy gave the player both the option of blaming a weak performance on the injury and afforded him elevated kudos within the club for his ability to play through pain and for his commitment to the club/team. A player's position in the club also counted. Howe detected a greater onus to 'deal with pain' when a player's position was under threat. As one player remarked to him:

> Since you have been around asking odd questions about my injuries and stuff I have really noticed how things have changed at the club. In the past I would 'cry-off' due to pain and minor injury, now my livelihood is dependent on performing well every Saturday. You have to suck it up in the modern era – hide the pain and play on'.

How vocal players were about pain was in fact contingent on assessments of costs and benefits:

> The mention of pain after a match could be used to save face when a player's performance was below par as a result of carrying an injury. Likewise when a player sustained a minor injury in training and could easily be replaced by another individual then there was a tendency to

conceal the pain and injury. On the other hand, a player who was a certain starter for every match, and much better than his understudies, would most likely do less to cover up the pain and injury that he might have been feeling. Such a player would not have wanted to cope with a pain that hindered his performance and in the long term impacted upon his chances of being the club's first-choice starter.

(Howe 2001: 295).

Assessments of this kind have been documented in other sports: see, for example, Huizenga (1994) on American football.

In Pontypridd RFC the severity of pain, Howe concludes, was always relative. Pain was a problematic marker for injuries. To many club officials, moreover, pain was not always a prime concern. Howe (2001: 298) again:

> in the professional era, when a winning team is paramount to a healthy balance sheet, the elimination of injury is all-important. The reduction in the amount of time needed to treat injury leads to team management getting more value for their money in relation to player contracts. This shift in treatment patterns, as a rapid return from injury becomes vital for the club, has left some long-serving members of the team concerned: 'In the past when I was injured I recovered at my own pace. Now it seems that my feelings about my fitness are not as important ... the club seems so concerned about getting their monies worth they have little time for me'.

Sport, health and identity

What these accounts indicate is the alarming extent and intensity of the pressures, many of them carrying high risks of injury, that attend opportunities for sporting success among one kind of contester, the professional rugby union player. But how do these accounts, and the discussion preceding them, bare on our principal theme of 'sport, health and identity'? It should be clear that whilst certain forms of moderate, rhythmic and regular exercise are likely to be protective of health, psychological as well as physical, many forms of sport are likely to be positively damaging to health. Moreover, the issue of identity – linked, as it is, to globalising tendencies, the reinvigoration of relations of class, processes of individualisation, the post-modernisation of culture and technologies of the self and governmentality – appears to be increasingly salient to the recasting of both exercise and sport in disorganised capitalism. But this needs unpacking.

It might plausibly be argued, first, that the search for a sustainable identity has become both more urgent and more volatile, disinhibited, and problematic in our post-modernised culture. As Bendle implies, analysts paradoxically see identity as having a novel, vital salience to individuals (his crisis of identity) at an historical juncture – the advent of the post-modern culture of disorganised capitalism – when identity formation is theorised as an ever more elusive, fluid and impermanent project (his crisis of 'identity'). Second, it might be contended that this is due in part to the prevailing culture-ideology of consumerism, itself the product of the resurgence of objective (if, paradoxically, not subjective) relations of class in the rapidly globalising era of disorganised capitalism. Health and sport, and the identities with which they have come to be associated, have grown more 'malleable', primarily as an unintended consequence of their (hyper)-commodification. In terms of health, this brings opportunities and hazards. On the positive side, people are freer to opt for, forge and be rewarded for identities through exercise and sport that are health-bestowing. On the negative side, as Monaghan's study shows, potentially health-bestowing activity can be subverted according to a formula implying that to look good is to feel good is to feel healthy. Sport is clearly not intrinsically healthy. Moreover, it is not unreasonable to contend that in disorganised capitalism the novel fluidity of identity-formation has permitted developments in sport that are objectively, if not subjectively, antithetical to health.

Amongst the contesters of professional rugby union, for example, the traditional ethos of 'manliness' has been given a new and harder edge. Of New Zealand rugby, Pringle (2001: 428) writes:

> the dominance of rugby helps circulate and promote knowledge that *real men* are tough and ignore pain. One result of this hypermasculine discourse is the large financial cost of rugby injuries. In the financial year 1997-98, the cost for rugby injuries was over $NZ25 million: including costs pertaining to two fatal injuries.

There is of course profit in this dominant discourse of manliness, which explains why the Maori *Haka* has been so comprehensively appropriated, 're-packaged' and exploited (Jackson and Hokowhitu 2002). But in an era of self-turnover, manliness is but one discourse, *petit* narrative or option for identity-formation.

Weiss (2001) draws attention to an interesting and pertinent paper by Popitz (1987) purporting to categorize people's demand for 'recognition' into five types of social subjectivity. It affords a framework to illustrate some of the themes of our discussion. The first type, 'recognition as member of a group', brings to mind Howe's account of the habitus of Pontypridd RFC, articulated through an intimate and closed network of symbolic rituals, encompassing wisecracks and horseplay as well as communication on the pitch. The second type Popitz terms 'recognition in an assigned role', referring to those self-affirming activities associated with, for example, gender: thus in rugby union masculinity is expressed through hard physical engagement and oblivion to pain, epitomised in what Pringle (2001: 431) calls 'perverse pleasures in the tackle'. The third type is 'recognition in an acquired role', incorporating both ability to perform a role (or role affirmation) and achievement beyond any potential present at birth. The kind of 'top performance' sought after by players in Ohlsson's and Howe's samples springs to mind here. 'Recognition in a public role' is Popitz's fourth type. Exemplars here are players who in Ohlsson's maximisation and pre-retirement phases make their marks in the public sphere, some even aspiring to become high-status, high-paid celebrities. Finally, the fifth type is 'recognition of personal identity'. The emphasis here is on individuality and difference. Ohlsson found that one way in which increasingly reflexive rugby players win a public role is through ensuring that they 'stand out' in team performances; and this might occur through a dramatic piece of play, for example a sidestep, try or tackle, or through an artefact like dyed hair. Implicit in Popitz's typology is the salience of recognition for identity-formation.

The contention of this chapter, in a nutshell, is that our post-modernised culture, characterised by a newly intense individualism, can only be explained sociologically with reference to the emergence of a culture-ideology of consumerism issuing from a reinvigoration of class relations concomitant with the global or disorganised capitalism of the last generation. These processes have facilitated Bendle's crises of identity and 'identity'. As far as sport is concerned, rather than finding themselves with more choices, people are increasingly seduced by the hypercommodification of either sport which is conducive to health or longevity or sport which is injurious to health and longevity. Moreover, the ends of health and longevity now represent one among many petit narratives. At the same time, people are increasingly attributed 'personal responsibility' for their health and longevity by the state via the mechanisms of technologies of the self and governmentality. There is, in other words, a price to pay for 'irresponsible' forms of seduction. As far as elite contesters like professional rugby players are concerned, the health cost can be high indeed. It may even be that such contesters, recognised and celebrated publicly by expedients like 'big hits', are the commodified products of a 'de-civilising spurt' in Elias' sense (see Elias Dunning 1986). The thesis that disorganised capitalism is witnessing such a de-civilising spurt deserves empirical attention. In the case of contemporary gladiators and gamblers, and perhaps paradigmatically quasi-legitimate 'no-holes-barred' or 'extreme fighting', redolent of the *pankration* of the ancient games at Olympia, the prima facie case seems well made. It was of the essence of Elias' figurational approach to modern sport that violence had been tamed by 'civilised' sensibility and ritual. A conjecture worth exploring across sport in high modernity, especially contact, combat and dangerous sports, is that violence is re-emerging in the form of commodified entertainment.

References

Beck U. (1992) *Risk Society: Towards a New Modernity*, London, Sage.

Bendle M. (2002) 'The crisis of "identity" in high modernity', *British Journal of Sociology*, 53 1–18.

Biddle S., Fox K. and Boutcher S. (2001) (eds) *Physical Activity and Psychological Well-Being*, London, Routledge.

Bourdieu P. (1977) *Outline of a Theory of Practice*, Cambridge, Cambridge University Press.

Bourdieu P. (1988) 'Programme for the sociology of sport' in S. Kang, J. MacAloon and R. DaMatta (eds) *The Olympics and Cultural Exchange*, Hanyang Ethnology Monograph 1, Hanyang, Hanyang University Press.

Bourdieu P. (1993) *In Other Words: Essays Towards a Reflective Sociology*, Cambridge, Polity Press.

British Medical Association (1992) *Cycling: Towards Safety and Health*, Oxford, Oxford University Press.

Donohoe T. and Johnson N. (1986) *Foul Play: Drug Abuse in Sports*, Oxford, Blackwell.

Dunning E. and Sheard K. (1979) *Barbarians, Gentlemen and Players: A Sociological Study of the Development of Rugby Football*, New York, New York University Press.

Eastbrooks P., Glasgow R. and Dzewaltowski A. (2003) 'Physical activity promotion through primary care', *Journal of the American Medical Association*, 289, 2913–16.

Elias N. and Dunning E. (1986) *Quest for Excitement*, Oxford, Blackwell.

Featherstone M. (1991) 'The body in consumer culture' in M. Featherstone, M. Hepworth and B. Turner (eds) *The Body: Social processes and Cultural Theory*, London, Sage.

Foucault M. (1979) 'On governmentality', *Ideology and Consciousness* 6, 5–22.

Foucault M. (1980) *Power/Knowledge*, Brighton, Harvester.

Gearing B. (1999) 'Narratives of identity among former professional footballers in the United Kingdom', *Journal of Aging Studies*, 13, 43–58.

Giddens A. (1990) *The Consequences of Modernity*, Cambridge, Polity Press.

Grant T. (2000) (ed.) *Physical Activity and Mental Health: National Consensus Statements and Guidelines for Practice*, London, Health Education Authority.

Hanson N. (1991) *Blood, Mud and Glory*, London, Pelham.

Held D., McGrew A., Goldblatt D. and Perraton J. (1999) *Global Transformations: Politics, Economics and Culture*, Cambridge, Polity Press.

Howe P. (1997) 'Commercialising the Body, Professionalising the Game: the Development of Sports Medicine at Pontypridd RFC' unpublished PhD thesis, University College London.

Howe P. (1999) 'Professionalism, commercialism and the rugby club: from embryo to infant at Pontypridd RFC' in T. Chandler and J. Nauright *The Rugby World: Race, Gender, Commerce and the Rugby Union*, London, Frank Cass.

Howe P. (2001) 'An ethnography of pain and injury in professional rugby union: the case of Pontypridd RFC' *International Review for the Sociology of Sport*, 36, 289–303.

Huizenga R. (1994) *You're Okay, It's Just a Bruise: a Doctor's Sideline Secrets about Pro Football's Most Outrageous Team*, New York, St Martin's Griffin.

Hume P. and Marshall S. (1994) 'Sports injuries in New Zealand: exploratory analysis', *New Zealand Journal of Sports Medicine*, 22, 18–22.

Jackson S. and Hokowhitu B. (2002) 'Sport, tribes and technology: the New Zealand All Blacks *Haka* and the politics of identity', *Journal of Sport and Social Issues*, 26, 125–39.

Klein A. (1993) *Little Big Men: Bodybuilding Subculture and Gender Construction*, New York, State University of New York Press.

Klein A. (1995) 'Life's too short to die small: steroid use among male bodybuilders' in D. Sabo and F. Gordon (eds) *Men's Health and Illness: Gender, Power and the Body*, London, Sage.

Korbut O. (1992) *My Story*, London, Century.

Lawlor D. and Hopker S. (2001) 'The effectiveness of exercise as an intervention in the management of depression: systematic review and meta-regression analysis of randomised controlled trials', *British Medical Journal* 322, 1–8.

Lyotard J.-F. (1984) *The Post-modern Condition*, Manchester, Manchester University Press.

Lynch J. and Carcasona C. (1994) 'The team physician' in B. Ekblom (ed) *Handbook of Sports Medicine and Science: Football (Soccer)*, Oxford, Blackwell Science.

Monaghan L. (2001) *Bodybuilding, Drugs and Risk*, London, Routledge.

Monaghan L. (2001a) 'Looking good, feeling good: the embodied pleasures of vibrant physicality', *Sociology of Health and Illness*, 23, 330–56.

Monaghan L. (2002) 'Vocabularies of motive for illicit steroid use among body-builders', *Social Science and Medicine*, 55, 695–708.

Morris J., Everitt M., Pollard R. and Chave S. (1980) 'Vigorous exercise in leisure time: protection against coronary heart disease', *Lancet*, 6 December, 1207–10.

Nepfer J. (1994) (ed.) *FIFA World Cup Report*, Zurich, FIFA.

Nettleton S. (1995) *The Sociology of Health and Illness*, Cambridge, Polity Press.

Paffenbarger R., Hyde R., Wing A. and Hsieh C. (1986) 'Physical activity, all-cause mortality, and longevity of college alumni', *New England Journal of Medicine*, 314, 605–13.

Popitz H. (1987) 'Autoritatsbedurfnisse: der wandel der sozialen subjektivitat', *Kolner Zeitschrift fur Soziologie und Sozialpsychologie*, 39, 633–47.

Pope H., Phillips K. and Oilivardia R. (2000) *The Adonis Complex: The Secret Crisis of Male Body Obsession*, New York, Free Press.

Pringle R. (2001) 'Competing discourses: narratives of a fragmented self, manliness and rugby union', *International Review for the Sociology of Sport*, 36, 425–39.

Rees P. (2003) 'Faster, fitter and so often fractured', The *Guardian*, 18 March.

Robertson R. (1992) *Globalisation: Social Theory and Global Culture*, London, Sage.

Royal College of Physicians (1991) *Medical Aspects of Exercise*, London, Royal College of Physicians.

Scambler G. (1996) 'The "project of modernity" and the parameters for a critical sociology: an argument with illustrations from medical sociology', *Sociology*, 30, 567–81.

Scambler G. (2001) 'Self-turnover, social representations and the culture-ideology of consumerism: a theory of self for the health domain', unpublished paper, Annual BSA Medical Sociology Conference, York, 22 September.

Scambler G. (2002) *Health and Social Change: A Critical Theory*, Buckingham, Open University Press.

Scambler G. (forthcoming) *Sport and Society: History, Power and Culture*, Buckingham, Open University Press.

Scott J. (2002) 'Social class and stratification in late modernity', *Acta Sociologica*, 45, 23–35.

Sklair L. (2000) 'The Transnational Capitalist Class', Oxford, Blackwell.

Smith A. and Jacobson B. (1988) (eds) *The Nation's Health*, London, King Edward's Hospital Fund for London.

Sports Council (1991) *Injuries in Sport and Exercise*, London, The Sports Council.

Sullivan S., Wong C. and Heidenheim P. (1994) 'Exercise related symptoms', *New Zealand Journal of Sports Medicine*, 22, 23–5.

Vincent J. (2003) *Old Age*, London, Routledge.

Waddington I. (2000) 'Sport and health: a sociological perspective' in J. Coakley and E. Dunning (eds) *Handbook of Sports Studies*, London, Sage.

Wallerstein E. (1998) *Utopistics: Or, Historical Choices of the Twenty-first Century*, New York, The New Press.

Wacquant L. (1995) 'Review article: why men desire muscles', *Body and Society*, 1, 163–79.

Weiss L. (1999) 'Managed openness: beyond neoliberal globalism', *New Left Review*, 238, 126–40.

Weiss O. (2001) 'Identity reinforcement in sport: revisiting the symbolic interactionist legacy', *International Review for the Sociology of Sport*, 36, 393–405.

Wilkinson R.G. (1996) *Health and Society: The Afflictions of Inequality*, London, Routledge.

Wittgenstein L. (1958) *Philosophical Investigations* (2nd ed.), Oxford, Blackwell.

Young K. (1993) 'Violence, risk and liability in male sports culture', *Sociology of Sport Journal*, 10, 373–396.

Young K., White P. and Mcteer W. (1994) 'Body talk: male athletes reflect on sport, injury and pain', *Sociology of Sport Journal*, 11, 175–94.

7

Lambegs and bódhrans: religion, identity and health in Northern Ireland

Ronnie Moore

Introduction

Northern Ireland is held by current Western world leaders (perhaps prematurely) as an exemplar of how peace can work. Since 1969 the Province has been synonymous with extreme social division. The basis of this lies in religious affiliation. A striking feature of Northern Irish society is that while religion may be seen as the generic cause of segregation and violence, community conflict is also tied in to inequalities, lifestyle, beliefs and wider notions of identity. While in a general sense Catholics and Protestants have a common culture in terms of sharing many of the basic features of modern living in the advanced industrial West, historical beliefs and practices operate to divide this small society. In addition there are other important nuances. Ethnic culture hinged around religious identity, influences social organisation and everyday life in profound ways. Importantly it can affect potential for assistance from family and friends and the willingness and ability to tap into important resources and information networks.[1]

This chapter discusses how this can significantly influence health. It is concerned with the connection between religion, identity and health, and presents findings from an ethnographic study of two small towns in Northern Ireland (one predominantly Roman Catholic and one Protestant). Key findings from the study are discussed and a number of themes are selected which illuminate the part religious differentiation plays in health and lifestyle issues. Finally, it summarises and draws the findings together within a unified theoretical framework.

Defining religion

The classic social science discussions on religion are summarised elsewhere (see, for example, Turner 1991). These place religion at the very centre of social life, social organisation and social behaviour. These belief systems or 'sacred canopies' codified and explained mystical and magical ideas that could not easily be understood or conceptualised, such as sickness and death, good and evil, luck and misery. For Malinowski (1948) these belief systems assumed important functions, 'helping to give structure and predict-ability to uncertain and dangerous contexts'. Magico-religious healing and reference to deities provided systems of coping with illness and distress (Turner 2000).

Durkheim underscored the important social basis of religion as represent-ing a common moral integrative value system with rituals, beliefs and prac-tices. Religion was an expression of 'collective social thought', shared experiences, and ideas about moral and social obligations (Durkheim 1976: 47). Weber was concerned with the social, political and economic consequences of religious formations and the effects of Calvinist doctrine stemming from the Reformation. Weber's interest was in the transformation from a Catholic Church dominated medieval Europe to the ascetic, com-petitive and rationalised ethic where individual, rather than the collective achievement, was emphasised (Weber 1958).

For Weber, Calvinist religion emphasised moral individualism, 'specifi-cally this worldly concerns for health and wealth', and the development of the Calvinist personality as crucially important to the rise of modern society (Turner 1991: 12).

I believe that we should regard the Protestant reformation as not only one source of modernisation, but also its defence against magic, superstition, witchcraft or mysticism. Calvinistic Protestantism was crucial in the devel-opment of modern forms of individuality, rationalism, and asceticism; it generated and preserved many of the essential features of what we mean by the notion of modernity. (Turner 1991: xvii).

It was this spirit which:

> contributed to the disciplined, this worldly-ethos of capitalist society by establishing vocational routines of hard work, calculation, and practic-ability.
>
> (Turner 1991: 28).

Health, social care and religion

The classic sociological texts from Comte through to Marx, Durkheim and Weber suggested that theistic aspects of religion would diminish in modern society. Indeed, as a belief system religion was certainly in crises throughout the nineteenth century as evolutionary and anthropological theories under-mined theological doctrine.

In the medieval period the church was central to healing and health care. The emergence of scientific rationalism, and the growth, expansion and dominance of scientific medicine throughout the last century essentially imposed themselves structurally, on modern life, and psychologically on modern thinking. These new paradigms attacked traditional ideas surrounding religion and consequently health and illness. Lay health beliefs and health practices, folk medicine and superstition were denigrated as sorcery or quackery. Yet we are reminded that modern medical and health services were inspired by and emerged from religious orders and monastic institutions (Lane 2001). Both family and church, even today, retain an important role as providers of health and social services in advanced industrial Western society and, as will be illustrated, play a part in the formation of identity.

Religion, culture and identity

Religion is an important marker for local, regional or national identity. The point is that religion is also an expression of a cultural system, and sense of belonging to a real or imagined community (Geertz 1966; Anderson 1983). As such it has consequences for social organisation, identity, physical and mental boundaries, a sense of belonging, language and expression, a sense of security, neighbourliness and co-operation, and conflict.

In Ireland, religion and the Christian church generally have played a significant role in establishing and regulating social, political, cultural, moral and psychological boundaries and social duties. Inglis (1998) provides an important summary of the religious 'habitus' of Irish Catholics, exploring the link between Irish nationalism and the Catholic collective conscience in what he describes as the Catholic churches 'moral monopoly'.

A potent representation of 'religion as culture', are the ethnic religious identities of Protestants and Roman Catholics who live in Northern Ireland, a politically contentious peripheral region of the United Kingdom. Religion and religious identity have been centre stage in what has euphemistically been referred to as, 'the troubles'. Northern Ireland, as a result, is often presented to the world as a dichotomous social structure with two competing ethnic religious groups with different national identities, British and Irish. The region is highly segregated (in the city and the country). More than 60 per cent of the population live in areas which have more than 80 per cent of one religion (O'Reilly and Stevenson 1998). This emphasises a high degree of homogeneity within these groups.

Northern Ireland is not only divided by religious sectarianism but also by social class, region and locality. There is strong identification and pride with local community. The effect of political violence serves to enforce the idea of group difference and has an influence on shaping identity within groups. It also militates against everyday interaction across the sectarian divide. Also, increasing long-term unemployment in Northern Ireland has meant that whole communities experience a more locally centred encapsulated and ghettoised lifestyle. Ties outside the local community are reduced with consequent effects on stereotyping, world view, political attitudes and the strength of boundaries. The boundaries are strongest in working-class areas, urban and rural.

'networks that cross the divide are largely based on pragmatic and uniplex relationships ... Multiplex ties are more likely in the case of professional classes ... In rural areas, these ties are the bases for co-operation between neighbours.

(Moore and Sanders 1996: 135).

However, this is often influenced by the security situation at the time.

The social and political aspects of Northern Ireland have long been dis-cussed and continue to be debated, health aspects less so. As a region it is characterised by low income, high levels of social deprivation, relative pov-erty, and (until recently) serious civil unrest (CSO 1994; London Health Economics Consortium 1995).

The cost of food, fuel and many other components of household expen-diture are higher than in the rest of the UK. Between 1993 and 1996 the number of families in receipt of one-parent benefit rose by 22 per cent. The proportion of people on attendance allowance, disability living allowance and incapacity benefit in Northern Ireland is twice as high as Great Britain. Almost one person in five over the age of 18 is on income support in Northern Ireland compared with one in eight in Great Britain (NISRA 1998).

Northern Ireland is a region with serious health concerns. It has dispro-portionately high levels of morbidity and mortality (especially in men). Circulatory and respiratory diseases such as ischaemic heart disease and cardiovascular illness are well documented (Barker *et al.* 1993). It has a higher average household size than the rest of the UK, a higher than average birth rate, and the number of single mothers has more than doubled since 1980. Women have the highest stillbirth rate and perinatal mortality in the UK, and there are significant variations in the incidence of low birth weights between electoral wards (Moore *et al.* 1997a).

Religion, identity and health: the research in Northern Ireland

National and international literature on health inequalities is now abundant and growing (Townsend, Davidson and Whitehead 1992). However, while Irish ethnic identity and the health of the Irish is now being addressed in Britain (Harding and Balarajan 1996; Abbotts *et al.* 1997; Kelleher and Hillier 1996; Abbotts, Williams and Smith 1999) and the USA (Kelleher *et al.* forthcoming), the lack of literature on the issue of religious identity and health *within* Northern Ireland is glaring (Campbell and Stevenson 1993).

Given the profile and importance of religious identity, politics, housing and employment in Northern Ireland, this lack of focus on religious affilia-tion and health is curious. Official research into medical and health care tended to concentrate on personal aspects of health, health related behaviour and service use, on structural, geographical and environmental accounts (and quantitative methods) and not religious/cultural ones.

In recognition of Northern Ireland's poor health record, the Department of Health and Social Services (DHSS) funded several recent research initiatives. In replicating the approach used by Townsend (1979), Stringer (1990) attempted to outline the severity and distribution of ill health and material deprivation in Northern Ireland, to account for inequalities in health, and to target health and areas of need. The analysis was at the geographical and electoral ward level, and it derived deprivation and health indices from the 1981 census data. It looked at the way, 'economic, social and environmental variables interact within small geographic areas so as to affect their populations' health'. The study mapped health variations on a province wide basis.

Campbell and Stevenson examined community differentials in self-reported health using the 1990/91 Continuous Household Survey. They reviewed available evidence on religious differences in health damaging behaviour and found few health differences between Catholics and Protestants (Campbell and Stevenson 1993). They noted a link between Catholic affiliation and smoking and also concluded that, while there were no significant differences between the proportion of Catholics and Protestants who drank alcohol, there were differences in the quantity of alcohol consumed by Catholics.[2] Catholic men were more likely to be classified as heavy drinkers.[3]

A subsequent report by Stringer (1992) did address religious affiliation and health. The basic findings are worth noting. For example, when using material deprivation and ward affiliation as a proxy, Stringer found an association between ill health and Catholic affiliation.

Further statistical analysis at sub-electoral ward level, however, pointed up more widespread geographic inequalities in mortality and morbidity than first thought. Indeed, controlling for deprivation it suggested higher ill health in some Protestant wards. Poorer health in Catholic wards was related to their poorer material condition rather than inherent differences in health status (Robson et al. 1994).

A summary of evidence on the nature and scale of health inequalities in Northern Ireland noted that:

> In income terms, similar proportions of Catholic and Protestant households live on very low incomes, but a substantially higher proportion of Protestants live on relatively high incomes than do Catholics.
>
> (London Health Economics Consortium 1995: 4).

The study suggested that materially deprived groups of Catholics and Protestants displayed 'correspondingly poor health status on the measures used', but that Catholic men appeared likely to smoke and drink more heavily than Protestants (London Health Economics Consortium 1995: 9).

Melaugh (1995) suggests that, strong cultural and group pressures are likely to influence smoking and drinking habits. This points to the influence of local cultural factors in health behaviour and lifestyle.

Crucially, the research concludes that 'wards which were overwhelmingly Catholic or overwhelming Protestant tended to display above average deprivation and ill health' (O'Reilly and Stevenson 1998: 167).

Background to the study

The government adopted a strategy to identify, target and reduce health inequalities and to provide equitable health care on a province-wide bases. In Northern Ireland much of the research into social and health inequalities has been statistical and epidemiological in nature and has tended to concentrate on income and deprivation as key to health status and health chances. These measured the associations between geographic, socio-economic and, environmental variables and health status and made inference to religious affiliation and health. The role religion and identity played in terms of promoting or negating health and well-being was not detailed. The interaction of local cultural and perceptual influences on the health experiences of individuals and groups at the local level were (and remain) largely neglected.[4]

Northern Ireland uniquely has integrated health and social care structures at department and health authority levels. The Department of Health and Social Services (DHSS) commissioned an ethnographic study of health and related need in two small rural communities in Northern Ireland (one predominantly Catholic/Nationalist and one predominantly Protestant/ Unionist). The study was designed to look at lay perceptions, issues and meanings of health in both rural communities, and at perceptions of health service delivery and health needs. The actual fieldwork phase was over a period of four months in each community. The rationale for the study, details on methodology employed, including choice of towns, is presented elsewhere (Moore et al. 1996). The research was fortuitously timed. The Provisional IRA and Protestant paramilitary cease-fire in the 1995–6 period meant that there was a more relaxed atmosphere in each of the communities, which facilitated the fieldworker's ingress to the community.

The findings of the research emphasised the multifactorial nature of the determinants of health and health behaviour and are presented in two government reports (Moore et al. 1997a/b). This short chapter presents a discussion of data that directly addressed issues of religion, identity and health. To provide some context for this it is important to review some of the key findings, and a brief discussion on selected issues is warranted.

Context of the study

The local economy for both small towns was mostly agricultural. These were very small market towns where sheep, cattle and dairy farming were important. In addition, there were usually small family-run businesses. In Ballymacross (Catholic), smallholdings were more common than in Hunterstown (Protestant) where farms tended to be bigger.[5] Unemployment was high in both towns. Throughout the 1980s and 1990s unemployment in Northern Ireland was growing faster in rural than in urban areas (Hart 1993). In the same period there was a dramatic decline in farming incomes. Many farmers, particularly in Ballymacross, supplemented their income by taking additional employment in construction (usually small building firms) or factory work or in services.

Marriage in both towns was traditionally endogamous. Intermarriage in Northern Ireland is infrequent. Close kinship shapes interaction in personal and private life, and lack of intermarriage restricts Protestant–Catholic interactions at the personal level. The tendency was to marry within the locality and remain geographically close to relatives. This meant that the communities were comprised of a number of long-standing, extended family groups. For other family members employment and life opportunities lay elsewhere and it was not unusual for several family members to live abroad temporarily or permanently (previously migration was usually to the USA but more recently England or the Irish Republic). This was especially true for Ballymacross.

Extended family groupings and 'friends' combined to determine the overall town membership: they were the reference point for defining individuals as insiders, i.e., coming from and being of the community, or 'blow-ins', (those who came from outside the town or local area).[6]

Ballymacross

Ballymacross was perceived principally as a Catholic town, although some Protestants lived in the surrounding area. It was located in mountainous picturesque landscape. The town was established around the mid-seventeen-hundreds by a land-owning family as a market centre for linen and livestock. The population was estimated to be just over one thousand. It was characterised by a settled, and fairly homogeneous community and was experiencing a recent rapid population increase by 47 per cent from 1981 to 1991. Dairy farming was practised, but since the land was poor, sheep farming was the primary source of agricultural income.[7] The introduction of quotas reduced the profitability of sheep farming resulting in many farmers taking additional work in other larger urban centres or in other small towns (Moore *et al.* 1997).

Most men were employed as skilled or semi-skilled wage labourers or farm labourers. A minority had their own small businesses in the form of small shops, garages or public houses. The town had recently received structural funding to 'kick start' regeneration, via property refurbishment and environmental improvement.[8] A local hotel had recently been renovated and provided work for a small number of local residents.[9] The principal shareholder and salaried staff however came from outside the town.

Catholicism was central to the religious, social and community life of Ballymacross. Active church attendance was almost universal. The church had a powerful influence in terms of regulating social life and social behaviour and enforcing rules at the local level. The education system was defined by the church and priests were actively involved in a range of social as well as religious events. The ethos emphasised family ties and community integration. There was no police station in the town. The role of the priest (from either of the two Catholic churches) extended to community policing when problems arose such as vandalism or theft, for example. Church life and community life in Ballymacross were strongly integrated. The provision of local church clubs and the Gaelic Athletic Association (GAA) reinforced links in the local community establishing them as separate even from other neighbouring Catholic towns.

Political, sporting and cultural interests tended to be similar in as much as they were in part determined by local cultural preference and by available resources. There was a small community centre, the small hotel and six public houses in the small town (and more in the immediate vicinity). The gaelic football, hurling and camogie teams were important in providing local sports opportunities. A Hibernian hall provided social events such as bingo, line dancing or fortnightly discos for various social groups. In addition, there were church-based craft groups and knitting groups.

There was no medical practice in Ballymacross. The nearest health centre was several miles away in a predominantly Protestant town. A central figure was the local pharmacist/chemist who was an important point of contact with the formal health care system and who provided a crucial health care service. This was partly because of the absence of a local doctor, partly because he was indigenous to the town and local culture and partly because of his ability as a local to understand and communicate with people in a personal, informal and discreet manner.

Hunterstown

Hunterstown was a predominantly Protestant town. It was settled originally in the seventeenth century mostly by Scots and English. Parish records refer to a wide range of occupations and growing prosperity during the industrial revolution. At the time of the study the population was around 1300. Farms tended to be bigger than in Ballymacross and the land tended to be better. It developed as a market centre for livestock and this was an important feature in the local economy. It also acted as an important service centre for out-lying hamlets and housing clusters in the hinterland. Applications for struc-tural funding by local councillors and community workers had been unsuccessful.

Close-knit family networks were an important feature in the town. However, the social structure of Hunterstown was more complex than that of Ballymacross. There was a high degree of social segmentation. Social class cleavages for example were more visible in Hunterstown. These were defined by wealth and social standing in the community, own-ership of farms, property, or commercial enterprises. Religious denomina-tion was also the source of social differentiation. The main churches included the Church of Ireland, Methodist, Presbyterian and Free Presbyterian and there were various other smaller Protestant sects, as well as Roman Catholics, who accounted for around 20 per cent of the local population (Moore *et al.* 1997a).

The various Protestant groupings had independent social/recreational net-works and some were more inclusive than others. The Free Presbyterians were perceived as being the most extreme and fundamental of all of the local denominations. One local Protestant commented:

> You couldn't talk to them. They've even got their own school and they have their own minibus to take kids to school. They are very closed and they all stick together. We are outsiders.
>
> (Sam, Hunterstown).

In addition, there were those who did not regard themselves as religious.

In Hunterstown, denomination and religiosity was perceived as a source of low-level division in two important ways. First, recreational activities were mostly church or school connected and (although sometimes denom-ination specific) almost totally religion specific. Second, there was a division between active churchgoers, those who attended occasionally, and those who did not attend. This had important resource consequences for non-churchgoers (although their children would often be members of church run clubs such as the Boys' Brigade). The lawn green bowling clubs were church run, as was the Women's Institute and a newly established children's playgroup. The newly formed photography club was, however, inde-pendent.

The Orange Institution was born in the local area. This is a pan-Protestant organisation which united local Protestants from various social back-grounds in defence against Catholicism and the threat of a united Ireland. The unity this identification afforded peaked at ceremonial high times such as the twelfth of July demonstrations/celebrations and similar events or at times of heightened political tension. In addition there was the Masonic Hall (although in a bad state of repair) used for very occasional social functions.

Unlike Ballymacross, Hunterstown had a health centre with several (male) physicians, district nurses and health visitors working from it. The role of the chemist contrasted with that of Ballymacross in that this was only one aspect of the total health care provision and not a principal feature of it.

Key findings from the study

While the link between socio-economic position and morbidity and mortality is now well established (Whitehead 1987; Townsend *et al.* 1992), this study emphasised that, over and above structural considerations, there was a complex interaction of influences on health and social well-being for both communities. In terms of key health issues, health perceptions and health problems, the similarities in both communities were more striking than observed differences (Moore *et al.* 1997a/b). Some of these are worth briefly noting.

Rural health experiences

Underlying structural influences impacted on health behaviour at several levels. Both towns suffered from high rates of unemployment, and were isolated from larger key centres and facilities. Hunterstown had better access to more immediate health care and treatment. However, many people registered with the doctors who lived outside the town. For local people from both towns the two key recurring issues were lack of local social/recreational facilities and poor transport. Local leisure and socialising activities for many in both towns were centred in public houses with limited appealing alternatives. In neither town was there a venue perceived as denominationally neutral for people to come together for recreation and community activities. The rural lifestyle was socially limiting and family, neighbour and church dependent. The strength of the collective identity in Ballymacross is illustrated:

> If anybody had to go to the hospital it's not a problem, because if you had no car, there's no problem asking somebody to run you anywhere. The place is that small and everybody knows everybody ... people would be offended it they thought you wouldn't ask them.
>
> (Maureen, Ballymacross)

Rural isolation featured prominently in both towns. Widespread feelings of isolation and depression particularly among women were related to confinement (often with children, but also with elderly kin) in the home, absence of social/recreational facilities or transport to reach facilities elsewhere, and the stress of managing a family on low income:

> There's a lot of carers in the area and they are not being treated properly at all ... Some of them aren't up to it. I mean, old men looking after their invalid wife, or *vice versa*, and their sons and children looking after aged parents, and women in their sixties looking after their mothers in their nineties, twenty four hours a day ... A letter from the Queen doesn't put food in your mouth or keep your house warm.[10]
>
> (Doris, Hunterstown).

In both towns individuals received health messages from health professionals but in many cases it was difficult to comply with recommended health behaviours. For example, physical exercise was encouraged but there were no accessible leisure centres. Mothers were advised to breast feed, but this was regarded as socially embarrassing and women who wanted to breast feed were often discouraged by the reactions of others, particularly men. This was true for both communities and health visitors reported an uphill struggle in trying to promote it (Moore *et al.* 1997a/b).

Alcohol and diet

Health behaviours were also embedded in local culture.[11] There was a marked drinking culture in both communities:

> There are two types of drinkers here, there's the hardened drinker and the alcoholic. Some people don't know which is which.
>
> (Joe, Hunterstown).

'Regulars' and publicans were neighbours and/or related, and the licensing laws were often flouted. The lack of local recreational facilities, the search for alternative venues in neighbouring towns, poor transport and local cultural peer pressure were cited as reasons for drunk driving. In Hunterstown there was also a strong anti-drink lobby.

Cheap convenience foods and the availability of more reasonably priced local meat and dairy produce, meant diets with a high fat content. Indeed, the 'Ulster fry', famous for its inclusion of meats and various other pan fried ingredients, was an important meal and was eaten for breakfast, at lunch time or in the evening.

Gender and health

In terms of gender, the health experiences of the two communities were similar. Strong family networks and neighbourliness in both towns operated not only as a system of social control but also crucially as a system of informal welfare in terms of Kleinman's (1993) well developed model. Women's identity was strongly linked to a maternal caring role. In terms of domestic health management, women took responsibility for the health of family members and made the decisions about what action to take when family members were ill. Men tended not to concern themselves with health issues. Younger mothers turned to their own mothers at times of crises and ill health, while older women depended on their daughters or other female kin. Even when it was necessary for a male relative to provide practical help, such as transport, it was often women who made the decisions.

In both communities, illness was perceived as weakness and doctor avoidance was prevalent. This had important implications, in particular for men's health and identity. Men were reluctant to admit to illness, consult doctors or take preventative measures, which were considered to be 'unmasculine'.

> My husband wouldn't go near the doctor unless he was really bad. I think most men are like that. I would nearly hold on and not go myself. You have to be bad before you see the doctor.
>
> (Bridget, Ballymacross).

> ... there is my husband and you just can't get him to go. I had to end up going to the doctor to tell him about it, but the doctor says that was no use, he would need to see it ... it would take the thing to be really showing on him before he would do anything about it.
>
> (Linda, Hunterstown).

Local health promotion strategies were set against this backdrop. This highlighted important health and information needs, which, although recognised by health professionals, were not adequately addressed.

Health beliefs

Beliefs about health were incorporated into an overarching fatalistic world view:

> If it happens to you it happens to you. You are going to die of something anyway, there's no point in worrying about it.
>
> (Robert, Hunterstown).

Another important point of similarity was the issue of lay healing. Strongly embedded in the local culture of both communities was the belief in what was locally called 'The Cure' or 'The Charm'. This is where a local person was identified as having a mystical gift of being able to provide a cure for a specific illness or for a variety of ailments. The oral tradition ensured its maintenance and reproduction. Many people were at some time taken to a healer or had chosen to seek out a cure or charm. Cures could be obtained for a variety of conditions ranging from minor complaints such as, sprains, tooth, stomach and headache, colic, various skin complaints, to the most serious conditions including cancers. The following narrative underlines the importance and centrality of informal healing in Ballymacross and Hunterstown.

> I have an open mind on charms because I have seen them work, both in my professional capacity and our private life ... the doctor said to me, 'you may go down and do the best you can for that man's got shingles ...', he [the man] said, 'Will you quit worrying nurse, I'm going for the charm tonight'. Quite honestly within a week he was completely healed and I couldn't see it in a month.
>
> (Madge, Hunterstown).

There were local sceptics in both communities, but a broad range of people talked about getting the cure. Teachers, health professionals, business people as well as ordinary people had gone for, or believed in the cure or charm. Folk medicine survived and co-existed symbiotically with the formal health system in both rural towns.[12]

Religion, identity and health experiences

The study also suggested important differences between the two communities. These were most noticeable in relation to ethnic religious identity, informal networks and support. Ballymacross was identified as a disadvantaged area and had received significant funding for regeneration. This prompted housing development and was said to have had a positive impact on the town. It became more attractive and 'a good place to live'. In contrast, Hunterstown was omitted as an area deserving of structural funding because outwardly, it looked more affluent. In the town and the wider rural area there were seams of extreme deprivation especially in specific housing clusters and satellite communities.

> OK, we do have affluence in this part of the world ... but if you are not in that bracket there is a big gap between those who are wealthy and those who are in poverty.
>
> (Albert, Hunterstown).

This highlighted the polarised nature (in terms of socio-economic status) of community life in Hunterstown. Class identity and class issues were an important feature in Huntertown narratives. The Hunterstown hotel, which had been derelict, was being rebuilt by a local builder, and one local man commented

> The hotel had a good effect on the town when it was there and it's being rebuilt. But again, it will be available to those who can afford it and maybe it will increase the social division, and the middle class will drink more in the hotel rather than the pubs.
>
> (Davy, Hunterstown).

The complex social structure in Hunterstown militated against community involvement or community action. The town was comprised of various groups, affiliations, and lifestyles and interests often differed considerably. Local people tended to interact with and rely on their immediate friends and relations and clearly defined social networks for advice, friendship and support. This in turn reinforced their identity. Feelings of marginality were expressed by less affluent residents.

> There hasn't been developing the sort of community infrastructure that exists in some other areas ... they are not seen as health issues, in fact, they are very important in terms of mental issues ... Mothers are trapped and access to cars is a big thing ... there is no recognition of the importance of these things.
>
> (Patricia, Hunterstown).

The effect of this was to increase the sense of relative deprivation. The perception was that:

> Catholics get everything, they know where to go and they have got good people working for them. We get nothing, there's nobody here does anything for us, you are just on your own, ... Even their clergy help them. Ours are useless ... see if ever you were in trouble you would never go to a Protestant councillor or solicitor. Their side work better for you ... Sure everybody knows that.
>
> (Gordon, Hunterstown).

Protestants in Hunterstown perceived Catholics to be tuned into to a culture of social interdependence and well established networks of information and support structures which helped them to access benefits more readily than Protestants. Catholics were seen as having better structures to deal with hardship and illness. They were seen as having a common spirit, close knit community support and close structural support from the Catholic Church and were seen as being concerted in their efforts in terms of providing mutual help. The perception was that while Catholics looked after their own people, Protestants looked after themselves as individuals. This, however, also depended on other factors as a local Catholic woman from Ballymacross suggests:

> I have lived fourteen years in Ballymacross ... It's a completely different culture from what I grew up and lived with [in Belfast] ... I found it very hard, very isolated, very much an invasion ... I found in Ballymacross there is a great inquisitiveness about yourself and who you were, and what you had done, and what land you had and what property ... Here it's all names. I found it very hard to adjust and the inquisitiveness and the unacceptability ... they didn't accept me ... At first I used to think it was me ... I get my full title, Mrs McGire when I go to the shop. I don't know half, quarter of the people here.
>
> (Bridie, Ballymacross).

In emergencies, Bridie could not access the same sort of support that her neighbours could.

> My son Michael had developed a limp ... I had to call the doctor out ... Dr Wilson had said to me on the phone, 'Could you run him in' [to the health centre] but my car was up at the mechanic ... I said I don't have a car. It wasn't an emergency, but the child was really in distress. He came out then.
>
> (Bridie, Ballymacross).

Support and identity did not solely rest on religion but also on 'belonging' (usually coinciding with religion). The social advantages which established Ballymacross people benefited from, were not necessarily extended to new-comers or perceived outsiders.

Catholic perceptions held that Protestants were generally economically more prosperous, with better land, better jobs, and bigger farms. At the local level, there was a degree of modesty and local people often talked down the sectarian. However, the general feeling was that Protestant history generally was one of colonial oppression and social, political and economic disenfranchisement:

> there's more of a class thing there ... they seem to have more. They have better shops and that.
>
> (Seamus, Ballymacross).

In Hunterstown, personal tensions such as social stigmatisation were also articulated. Catholics have this communal thing ... In the Protestant community you see, you don't want to stand out ... there would be a fair amount of stigma ... I mean you hear comments about getting free school meals.

> (Davy, Hunterstown).

The expectation was to conform to your own principles of social behaviour that included being independent and self-reliant.

> Those one's who get involved, get involved in everything. You would see the same faces at everything.
>
> (Brenda, Hunterstown).

Catholics were seen to be able to access wider social resources without fear of stigmatisation. The collective identity allowed for this.

Social stigma, lack of information and support groups were important issues for local people in both communities, but these appeared to be much more acute in Hunterstown. Also, conceptualising illness as weakness had wider consequences. Health visitors and local doctors defined asthma as a major and growing problem among children in the wider area and an asthma clinic was established in Hunterstown. However, mothers were reluctant to bring their children to it because of the social stigma attached to the condition.

> People are very funny about asthma, they get upset, annoyed and even cross if you suggest that their child has asthma.
>
> (Peter, primary school principal near Hunterstown).

In Ballymacross, local people collectively attached importance to their local culture and Catholicism. As an institution the Catholic church centrally underpinned moral and social living in Ballymacross. Important demonstrable examples of social and health benefits of living in Ballymacross included sensitive treatment of those on the economic and social margins, including local alcoholics, older people living alone and those with mental health problems.

Helpful information networks were more readily identified in Ballymacross.[13] The moral obligation to show an awareness and understanding of those in difficult social or health circumstances was emphasised by the response of local people who actively engaged with a man with visible mental health problems:

> That's Patrick, he's got a few mental problems like ... You might have seen him at the hotel ... he's usually there at lunch times ... If nobody's here, Gerry [the bar man] or somebody usually sorts his money out [payment] for him ... He's a harmless sort.
>
> (Damien, Ballymacross).

Patrick's mental health problems were known by many, and he experienced direct and indirect support even from what might be regarded as unlikely quarters. For example, local young men in various contexts afforded him courtesy and assistance. Provision was made in a local pub for him to come for his lunch (usually free) and local people, even though he may not have been directly included in their company, kept a careful watch and assisted him. The strength and value of this collective spirit was widely recognised:

> In the city people with disabilities are ignored a bit more. Here we would care for them ... maybe a neighbour would help.
>
> (Karen, Ballymacross).

Patrick's experience was not isolated.

Social isolation and health

Restricted transport was the single major barrier to access to health, social and recreational facilities. In Ballymacross while local people saw the remoteness of the health centre as an inconvenience most did not regard this as a major problem. This pointed up transport and use of a car as a rural necessity in both communities. As such it was deemed an important feature in terms of access to health (often *inaccurately* calculated as a key proxy indicator for socio-economic and thus health status).

The sense of powerlessness was particularly expressed and articulated in Hunterstown. Social isolation and lack of community integration were considered to be negatively influencing factors:

> ... it prevents people going and seeking support and seeking some kind of counselling. In my experience people internalised issues such as abuse and that kind of thing. Women feel they have to put up with what they have got ...
>
> (Madge, Hunterstown).

Post Natal Depression (PND) was a case in point. Some women interviewed in both areas said they had experienced PND and expressed feelings of extreme emotional anxiety. Women reported a lack of adequate formal medical support structures. Local doctors, and even women's partners were perceived as not fully appreciating their illness. Social stigmatisation, rural isolation and being seen as not being able to cope were repeatedly articulated. Women reported that even basic information was not available.

The experience in Hunterstown meant that women relied more on informal support via the immediate family and less on extra familial support, which was more often the case in Ballymacross. One sufferer suggested providing special training to help partners and family understand and cope with PND.

> My depression was not diagnosed by the doctors. Every time I went, they kept giving me these creams and rubs and things. They didn't pick

up on it. They were looking for something physically wrong with me and not mentally... it might have been easier if there was a woman doctor there. I really don't know if they understand.

(Barbara, Hunterstown).

Religion, location and disadvantage

Relatively small numbers of Catholics lived in Hunterstown, and even fewer Protestants lived in Ballymacross. There were two important aspects to this. It was perceived to be more advantageous for Protestants living around Ballymacross (if necessary) to tap into the local resources such as the credit union, even the 'St Vincent de Paul society' and in social and cultural events such as Irish music festivals. There was scope for inclusivity in these events and services. Protestant mores and fear of surveillance however, often (but not always) militated against it.

It's a dignity thing ... people round here talk.

(Jean, Ballymacross).

However, Catholics living in Hunterstown appeared to fare worse in terms of utilising networks and social support because existing community resources (limited as they were for Protestants) provided even less for them:

There's no St Vincent de Paul, no Help the Aged, no Save the Children in Hunterstown. But they have their own credit union now and the Orange Order have their own one.

(Clare, Hunterstown).

In contrast to Ballymacross, Catholics in Hunterstown felt isolated and fragmented and their social networks were extremely limiting. One Catholic man from Hunterstown states:

I think Catholics are quite happy being insular ... your neighbour could be Catholic or non-Catholic. They don't really mix ... We had an interview with a journalist in the summer there ... and one's [local Protestants] were saying that it's no problem at all. But that's not true. We would find that we are polarised to the bottom end of the town ... but again that's historic, that's where our people went to live.

(Kieran, Hunterstown).

Protestants in Hunterstown felt they had good social relations with Catholic neighbours who lived in or around the town and considered Catholics in the town to be well integrated. This perception was not always shared by

Catholics themselves. Catholics in Hunterstown felt isolated and alienated from many aspects of social life.

There was a marked contrast in the general morale and outlook of the respective populations. Ballymacross was a growing, thriving town which had experienced regeneration. There was a strong identification with community which had been reinforced by collective interest in regeneration projects. In contrast, people in Hunterstown felt 'forgotten about':

> The people in Hunterstown are so used to having nothing that they have come to accept it as a way of life. But if you stand back and look at other areas, it's obvious just how hard done by we are here. The place has actually been nicknamed 'the forgotten town' ... it's not a healthy environment for children.
>
> (Cheryl, Hunterstown resident and doctor).

The communal spirit which was talked up in Ballymacross was confined to disparate groups in Hunterstown. Belonging to the Unionist tradition was a unifying feature for most people in terms of Protestant identity and opposition to a Catholic dominated united Ireland, although explicit expression of this was only intermittent through seasonal Protestant celebrations such as orange parades and marches. The spirit was neither enduring nor complete. The community was sub-divided by religion (main denominations and various sects) and the 'good living', by social class, and those who were 'non religious'.

Religion and risk

Religion was also an important determinant of risk factors in terms of common and serious rural accidents. On the larger farms (more common in Hunterstown) there were specific risks. Just prior to the study a young child had suffocated in a grain pit. During the fieldwork two young brothers who worked on the family farm died when they were overcome by toxic fumes and fell unconscious into a slurry pit.

In Ballymacross, primary care was more remote than in Hunterstown. While most farmers from large farms attended agricultural college and were aware of formal requirements and regulations on health and safety measures, this was not the case for small or part time (hobby) farmers who were less likely to receive formal agricultural education nor were their farms formally inspected. One young man from Ballymacross had lost the use of three of his fingers as a result of an accident with an engine. He did not present to the doctor for a considerable period.[14] This stoicism was a feature of male identity in both communities.

Discussion

The research suggests that although the construction of health and the health experiences of both communities are in very many ways similar, there are also important nuances. These hinge on religious affiliation and have consequences for physical and mental health and well-being.

Religion and local identity in Northern Ireland prescribe a world view and concomitant social action. This is sustained by enduring moral and ethical ways of thinking and acting. Bourdieu refers to this as 'habitus'. For Bourdieu 'structure determines the perceptual boundaries underlying choice and this is critical in health lifestyle selection' (Bourdieu 1984). Habitus means that a person does not necessarily need to be religious *per se* to feel compelled by social stigma, local mores and moral obligations. Ethical principles (and political identity) were commonly assigned by virtue of religious affiliation.

In Ballymacross and Hunterstown, structure, religion and local culture oriented habitus influenced health lifestyles, health chances and health risk. Individuals' health-promoting opportunities and decisions, were guided by religious affiliation and local cultural principles. This enabled or inhibited social support networks and information. Established Ballymacross residents tended to have and utilise wide and often well established social and information networks (although the extent and quality of these networks were often over stressed by Protestants), whereas in Hunterstown these tended to be restricted to more immediate networks. Drum making may be seen as an important, if ironic, metaphor in this regard. A Hunterstown drum maker said that 'bódhran' drum makers frequently contacted him to buy skin off-cuts and they now copy the 'lambeg' drum making process of curing drum skins.[15]

The concept of social capital is also important to health and health chances. Recognition of the part social capital plays in health is now well established and debated (Putnam 1993/95; Campbell *et al.* 1999; Kawachi and Kennedy 2002). Social capital refers to the rules that reflect community values and norms and which provide for various coping strategies, durable networks, marriage, kinship networks, extra familial support structures and secular and religious community institutions. It is the cumulative totality of all of the resources available to individuals through their social affiliations and membership. This could include passing on second-hand clothes, to babysitting, to information exchange, to basic interaction.

The particular modes of social organisation in Northern Ireland are an adaptive response to a political identity; religious ethic; sectarian segregation; and pragmatic living. While socio-economic position was considered a major influence affecting health and life chances, culture and religious habitus influenced social living and health in small but profound ways. Personal choices and health chances are contingent upon conditions such as social

class, but religious beliefs and religious affiliations were an important orga-
nising principle affecting the health lifestyles of both communities. Ethnic
religious identity provided the basis for social capital potential and this
works at different physical spheres, domestic, town, locality, and beyond.[16]
The difference between Ballymacross and Hunterstown is the degree of and
scope for social capital potential. Both encapsulated communities recognised
this and knew the operating structures and cultural limitations emphasised
by their respective communities.[17]

Ballymacross was seen as supporting a unified Catholic ethos and identity
with the strict involvement of religion and the church. Religion and religiosity were central, in terms of local identity and national allegiance, and the
church was actively engaged in social living at various levels – local policing,
therapeutic listening and administering advice, as well as providing support
for social, cultural and sporting events.

Hunterstown reflected not only historical denominational divisions, but
also more recent fundamentalist factions in the form of new (inspirational)
Protestantism or new church groupings such as the Free Presbyterians
(Bruce 1986; Moore and Sanders 2002).

For Weber, independence (evangelical freedom and personal piety),
autonomy and destiny constituted a necessary ideological condition for
the success of early capitalism. Calvinism emphasised asceticism and personal success as important for salvation. But capitalist success and the
Protestant principle of subjectivism (*sola fide*) has undermined religious
meaning, has made Protestantism essentially fissile, and has been a source
of community division. A unified Protestant doctrine does not exist and is
not practised (in contrast to Roman Catholic doctrine). Calvin, for example,
emphasised the doctrine of predestination; other fundamental evangelical
sects emphasised salvation through being 'born again'. The various
Protestant churches and sects respectively provide support basis for their
members and enforce their own brand of social inclusion and social control.

As Bruce suggests, traditional Protestant denominations have experienced
decline over the last century with disaffected Protestants turning to conservative churches such as the Free Presbyterian church and to fundamental Protestant sects (Bruce 1983). In addition, liberal Protestantism has
encouraged the tendency towards secularisation. For Protestants there is
no one unified church and no overarching moral authority. Protestant
formations compete against each other (as well as Catholicism), with
secularisation, and struggle with the effects of late capitalism. This has
implications in terms of identity and cohesion and translates into health
issues. In contemporary capitalism moral individualism is a cause of dis-
enchantment, confusion and 'anomie' among Protestants in Hunterstown.[18]
It translated into atomised groups with competing interests, fatalistic
attitudes, feelings of relative deprivation and powerlessness to compete
with effects of globalisation.

For Catholics in Ballymacross the church is the single unifying feature in terms of identity. This has endured through the reformation, land dispossession, famine and imperialism. Catholicism provides community leadership, direction and therapeutic communication (auricular confession) through priests. The distinctive symbolic rituals and icons central to Catholicism remain central. A major hallmark is a unified, universal doctrine emphasising social and moral values and religious and political obedience. For local people in Ballymacross Catholicism equates to culture, identity, social control, social cohesion and social welfare. It is social cement. In Ballymacross an egalitarian Catholic ethos culturally produced social/health capital and promoted well-being, for established local people. This contrasts with Hunterstown where the ethos for many was personally and socially restrictive and was suggestive of Weber's concept of 'inner loneliness' as the consequence of the Calvinist ascetic lifestyle and Protestantism on identity choices (Gerth and Mills 1946).

Those in the most vulnerable position of all were Catholics living in Hunterstown who expressed a greater degree of physical and social isolation than their Protestant neighbours.

Conclusion

The government in Northern Ireland has now a strategic interest in 'bottom up' approaches to dealing with health and health care and in how and to what degree aspects of health are mediated within communities at the local level. This study suggests that social capital importantly influences other forms of capital such as health capital. It also raises a number of issues in relation to ethnic identity and health. Conceptualisation of a dichotomous split solely along ethnic religious lines in Northern Ireland is seen as problematic on several counts. It assumes a static homogeneity and separateness within the two dominant religious groups. However, high and low level fragmentation was evident within both communities studied, but particularly within Hunterstown. Research has hitherto ignored other fluid, hybrid and contingent forms of identity (for example, co-religionists who lived in, but were not from Ballymacross, who expressed feelings of exclusion and isolation). Also, the health issues of other ethnic groups in Northern Ireland (such as the Chinese and Asian communities), traditionally overlooked, have only recently been addressed (Hainsworth 1998).[19]

References

Abbotts J., Williams R., Ford G., Hunt K. and West P. (1997) 'Morbidity and the Irish Catholic descent in Britain: An ethnic religious minority 150 years on', *Social Science Medicine*, 45, 3–14.

Abbotts J., Williams R. and Smith G.D. (1999) 'Association of medical, physiological, behavioural and socio-economic factors with elevated mortality in men of Irish heritage in West Scotland', *Journal of Public Health Medicine*, 21, 1, 46–54.

Anderson B. (1983) *Imagined Communities: Reflections on the origin and spread of Nationalism*, London, Verso.

Barker M., McLean S. and McKenna P. (1993) *Diet, Lifestyle and Health in Northern Ireland: A Report to the Health Promotion Trust*, Coleraine, University of Ulster.

Bourdieu P. (1984) *Distinctions*, Cambridge, MA, Harvard University Press.

Bruce S. (1986) 'The Persistence of religion: Conservative Protestantism in the United Kingdom', *Sociological Review*,31.

Campbell R. and Stevenson G. (1993) *Community Differentials in Health in Northern Ireland*, Belfast, Department of Health and Social Services.

Campbell C., Wood R. and Kelly M. (1999) *Social Capital and Health*, London, Health Education Authority, Trevelyan House.

Central Statistical Office (1994) *General Household Survey*, 29 (101), London, HMSO.

Cockerham W., Abel T. and Lüschen G. (1993) 'Max Weber, Formal Rationality, and Health Lifestyles', *Sociological Quarterly*, 34, 3, 413–28, in W. Cockerham (ed.) (1995) *The Sociology of Medicine*, Aldershot, Edward Elgar.

Durkheim E. (1976 [original 1915]) *Elementary Forms of Religious life*, London, Allen and Unwin.

Friel S., Nic Gabhainn S. and Kelleher C. (1999) *Results of the National Health and Lifestyle surveys, Slan and HBSC*, Galway, Centre for Health Promotion Studies.

Geertz C. (1966) 'Religion as a cultural system' in M. Banton (ed.) *Anthropological approaches to the study of Religion*, London.

Gerth H.H. and C. Wright Mills (trans. and ed.) (1946) *From Max Weber: Essays in Sociology*, New York, Oxford University Press.

Greer J. and Murry M. (eds) (2003) *Rural Planning and Development in Northern Ireland*, Dublin, Institute of Public Administration.

Greenslade L. (1995) 'A good man's fault: Alcohol and Irish people at home and abroad', *Alcohol and Alcoholism* 30, 4, 407–17.

Hainsworth P. (1998) Divided Society: Ethnic Minorities and Racism in Northern Ireland, London, Pluto.

Harding S. and Balarajan R. (1996) 'Patterns of mortality in second generation Irish living in England: Longitudinal Study', *British Medical Journal*, 312: 1389–92.

Hart M. 'Enterprise in Rural Areas' in M. Murray and J. Greer (eds) (1993) *Rural Development in Ireland*, Aldershot, Avebury.

Inglis T. (1998) *Moral Monopoly: The rise and fall of the Catholic Church in Modern Ireland*, Dublin, University College Dublin Press.

Inglis T. 'Catholic Church religious Capital and Symbolic Domination' in M. Böss and E. Maher (eds) (2003) *Readings of Politics culture and Literature at the Turn of the Century*, Dublin, Veritas

Kawach I. and Kennedy B. (2002) *The Health of Nations: Why inequality is harmful to your health*, New York, New Press.

Kelleher D. and Hillier S. (1996) The Health of the Irish in England. Researching Cultural Differences in Health, London, Routledge.

Kelleher C.C., Harper S.H., Lynch J.W., Tay J.B. and Nolan G. (forthcoming) 'Hurling Alone: How Social Capital failed to save the Irish from Cardiovascular disease in the United States of America', *American Journal of Public Health*.

Kelleher C., Hope A., Barry M. and Sixsmith J. (2001) *Health, safety and well being in Rural Communities in the Republic of Ireland: Main Results from the Agriproject. Centre for Health Promotion Studies*, Galway, National University of Ireland.

Kleinman A. (1980) *Patients and Healers in the Context of Culture*, Los Angeles, University of California Press.

Lane J. (2001) The Social History of Medicine: Health, healing and disease in England 1750–1950, London, Routledge.

London Health Economics Consortium (1995) *Health and Social Inequality in Northern Ireland: Factors influencing the development and implementation of policy towards reducing inequality in health – Lessons from the International Experience*, report to the DHSS, London, London School of Hygiene and Tropical Medicine.

Melaugh M. (1995) 'Majority–minority differentials: unemployment, housing and health' in Dunn S. *Facets of Conflict in Northern Ireland*, London, Macmillan.

Malinowski B. (1948) *Magic, Science and Religion*, Boston, MA, Beacon.

Moore R. and Sanders A. (1996) 'The limits of an anthropology of conflict, Loyalist and Republican paramilitary organisations in Northern Ireland' in A. Wolfe and H. Yang (eds) *Anthropological Approaches to Conflict Resolution*, Athens, Georgia.

Moore R., Mason C., Harrisson S. and Orr J. (1996) 'The use of an ethnographic approach to assessment of health need in Northern Ireland', *Nursing Times Research*, 1, 4, 252–8.

Moore R., Harrison S., Mason C. and Orr J. (1997a) *An assessment of Health inequalities in Two Northern Ireland Communities: An Ethnographic Approach*, report for the Department of Health and Social Services in Northern Ireland, Belfast, The Queen's University of Belfast.

Moore R., Harrison S., Mason C. and Orr, J. (1997b) *Health Professionals' Perspectives on Service Delivery in Two Northern Ireland Communities*, report for the Department of Health and Social Services in Northern Ireland, Belfast, The Queen's University of Belfast.

Moore, R. and Sanders A. (2002) 'Formations of Culture: Nationalism and Conspiracy Ideology in Ulster Loyalism', *Anthropology Today*, 18, 6, 9–15. London, Blackwell.

Mullen K., Williams R. and Hunt K. (1996) 'Irish decent, religion, and alcohol and tobacco use', *Addition*, 91, 2, 243–54.

Northern Ireland Statistics and Research Agency (1998) *Regional Trends for Northern Ireland*, Belfast, Department of Economic Development.

O'Reilly D. and Stevenson M. (1998) 'The Two Communities in Northern Ireland: Deprivation and ill health', *Journal of Public Health Medicine*, 20, 2, 161–8.

Putnam R. (1993) 'The Prosperous Community: Social Capital and Public Life', *American Prospect*, 13: 35–42.

Putnam R. (1995) 'Bowling Alone: America's Declining Social Capital', *Journal of Democracy*, 6, 1, 65–79.

Rivers W.H.R. (1924) *Medicine, Magic and Religion*, New York, Harcourt Brace.

Robson B., Bradford M. and Deas I. (1994) *Relative Deprivation in Northern Ireland*, Policy Planning Research Unit, Belfast, Department of Finance and Personnel.

Stringer P. (1990) *Spatial and social variations in the distribution of health indictors in Northern Ireland*, Policy Research Institute, Department of Health and Social Services in Northern Ireland, Belfast, The Queen's University of Belfast.

Stringer P. (1992) *Health Inequalities, religious affiliation and urban – rural status*, Policy Research Institute, Department of Health and Social Services in Northern Ireland, Belfast, The Queen's University of Belfast.

Turner B. (1991) *Religion and Social Theory*, London, Sage.

Turner B. in Albrecht G., Fitzpatrick R. and Scrimshaw S. (eds). (2000) *The handbook of Social Studies in Health and Medicine*, London, Sage.

Townsend P. (1979) *Poverty in the United Kingdom*, London, Penguin.

Townsend P., Davidson, N. and Whitehead, M. (1992) *Inequalities in Health: The Black Report – The Health Divide*, London, Penguin.

Weber M. (1958) *The Protestant Ethic and the Spirit of Capitalism*, New York, Schribner.

Whitehead M. (1987) *The health divide: Inequalities in health in the 1980s*, London, HEA.

Wilkinson R.G. (1996) *Health and Society: The Afflictions of Inequality*, London, Routledge.

Notes

1. In Northern Ireland the term 'tap' also refers to asking for money.
2. Mullen, Williams and Hunt (1991) provide a useful discussion on religious affiliation and tobacco and alcohol use in the West of Scotland.
3. Yet research in the Republic of Ireland noted significant proportions of people who said they did not drink alcohol (see Friel S., Nic Gabhainn S. and Kelleher C. 1999).
4. Recent studies attempting to account for ethnic religious health differences remain epidemiological in approach. A 'descriptive "epidemiological study" suggests that Catholic areas appear to be more disadvantaged than Protestant areas.' The authors however concede that, 'in Northern Ireland it is possible to select an indicator which will support any previously held prejudice'. They conclude that there was much more variability within Catholic and Protestant areas than between them. (O'Reilly and Stevenson 1998: 166).
5. In order to preserve confidentiality Ballymacross and Hunterstown are pseudonyms.
6. 'Friends' in the Irish sense often indicates an affinity. Distant relatives are usually referred to as 'a friend'.
7. The land nearer the mountains was not as easily worked as the low lands. This meant that there was little clearance of the native population according to the 1659 census.
8. Ballymacross was awarded £998,000 by the International Fund for Ireland and the Department of Environment (NI). The money was to be used to improve the appearance of the town, rebuild the old hotel and create a new resource from the former Protestant primary school.
9. Under the auspices of Community Regeneration and Improvement Special Programme (CRISP).

10. In Britain and Northern Ireland when a person reaches the age of one hundred they traditionally receive a letter of congratulations from the Queen.

11. The literature is complex here. Research elsewhere suggests little observed difference between Irish and English drinking patterns although the Irish appear to consume greater amounts of alcohol (Greenslade 1995). Recognition of widespread and excessive drinking as a social problem came in recent comments made in the USA and Ireland by the President of the Irish Republic and the Irish government have recently introduced measures to curb what they see is a major social issue.

12. Going for a cure took pressure off overburdened physicians and health care professionals. Curers differed significantly from 'faith healers' for example, the seventh son (or daughter) or the seventh son of the seventh son (See for example, Buckely 1981, Moore *et al.* 1997a). The gift of the cure was assigned to the healer on the bases of birthright, inheritance or some other circumstances. For example, it was commonly believed that someone who was born after the death of the father automatically assumed the cure for oral thrush or 'badmouth' irrespective of whether the father had the cure. The practical act of curing varied. It could involve a laying of hands on affected parts of the body, prayers, the use of sticks and/or specially prepared substances. People with the cure did not choose to have it. It was bestowed on them and they chose to keep it and use it or not. Some were reluctant practitioners driven by a sense of responsibility rather than by personal choice. Curers did not ask for, nor necessarily accept monetary payments for their services. They might accept payment in kind.

13. These also extended to networks abroad.

14. Similar issues were subsequently reported in research in the Republic of Ireland (see for example, Kelleher C., Hope A., Barry M. and Sixsmith J. 2001).

15. The bódhran is a small drum culturally associated with Irish traditional music, while the lambeg drum is a very large drum which is a symbol of Protestantism in Northern Ireland.

16. Inglis (2003) offers an important discussion on religious capital.

17. Health capital has hitherto been less articulated as an additional form of capital.

18. Durkheim introduced 'anomie' as a failure of moral regulation when individual interests and personal desires and power go unregulated.

19. The travelling community, the Asian and the Chinese community received little attention. This has only been addressed in recent research.

8

Gay and lesbian identities and mental health

Michael King and Eamonn McKeown

Lesbians and gay men are a significant but mainly invisible minority in Britain. Five per cent of men and 3 per cent of women report that they have had some 'homosexual experience' in the preceding five years (Sell *et al.* 1995). In major cities, the population is much bigger, for example in Greater London up to 12 per cent of men report sexual relationships with other men (Johnson *et al.* 2001). This constitutes around $2\frac{1}{4}$ million people in Great Britain. Little is known about the relationship between self identification as gay or lesbian and psychological health or social well being. Self identity in gays and lesbians is complex and there is no universal language in which it is expressed (Cabaj and Stein 1996). Individuals who define themselves as gay or lesbian form a group whose life-style may differ from the dominant culture. However, the public profile of the gay 'scene' touches only a tiny proportion of gay and lesbian people who move within a certain commercial culture.

Defining same sex attraction

Kinsey's famous studies in the United States in the 1940s rated individuals on a seven-point scale according to their life-time homosexual and heterosexual experiences. This excluded those with homosexually oriented fantasy and took little account of self-identification (McWhirter *et al.* 1990). In their national study of sexual behaviour in Britain, Wellings *et al.* (1996) did not include the term homosexual in their questions. They held it to be stigmatising and medicalising. Instead, individuals were asked to rate themselves on attraction to and sexual experience with same and opposite sex partners on a six-point scale. There is more to being gay or lesbian, however, than sexual behaviour with people of the same gender. Of equal importance is individuals' identity as gay/lesbian (homosexual), bisexual or straight (heterosexual). This will more often determine their lifestyle and how others react to them than a reductionist view of their sexual behaviour. Gay people live in a variety of ways from outwardly as heterosexuals with spouses and children to individuals who identify exclusively with a commercial gay subculture.

Homosexuality as mental pathology

There are many positive aspects to being gay. Lesbians and gays may be more resourceful and self-reliant, have a wider circle of supportive friends and more disposable income than heterosexuals. Nevertheless, homosexuality remains a stigmatised concept (Saad 1998) that was until relatively recently used as a diagnostic term in international psychiatric diagnostic glossaries (Spitzer 1981). Official sanction of homosexuality as illness distorted any development of gay and lesbian identity and led to oppression, shame, guilt and fear for many men and women and their families. Over many decades in the twentieth century, gay men in particular underwent psychoanalytical and psychiatric treatments to become heterosexual that had major negative effects on their sense of identity, self esteem, mental health and well-being (King and Bartlett 1999; Smith *et al.* 2003; King *et al.* 2003). Gay men and lesbians with psychological difficulties continue to be treated mainly by heterosexual psychotherapists and psychiatrists, whose theoretical training has been, by today's standards, homophobic (Bartlett *et al.* 2001). In the United States, so-called reparative therapy continues to be promoted by religiously orientated professionals and by psychoanalysts who hold entrenched views that homosexuality can be cured (Haldeman 1994; Drescher 1998). How common such practice is in Britain is unknown. However, negative views of gays and lesbians are held by medical students (Evans *et al.* 1993; McColl 1994) and health (Bhugra and King 1989; Rogers 1998) and mental health care professionals (McFarlane 1997). Teaching about gay and lesbian issues in medical schools is in its infancy (Bewley 1997).

Mental health and a gay identity

Gay people are disadvantaged in modern society and may be vulnerable to mental disorders. Even in our arguably more liberal, modern society, prejudice remains common in personal and public life. Unlike people from ethnic minorities, gays and lesbians can blend with the heterosexual majority, but at the psychological and social cost of hiding their identity and lifestyle from friends and even family. Furthermore, they have no recourse to legal protection from discrimination. Gay men and lesbians do not have equal rights with heterosexuals in terms of age of consent to sexual activity, marital relationships, next of kin issues, pension rights, care and control of children, or the right to serve in Her Majesty's Armed Forces. Fortunately, the British government has just published a white paper that proposes redress in these areas by recognising same-sex, civil partnerships (http:// www.dti.gov.uk/consultations/pdf/consult-civil.pdf).

Ethnic minority gay men and lesbians exist as minorities within minorities and must bear multiple levels of discrimination (Greene 1994). Growing up having to conceal one's sexual development and often being exposed to hostility, may have had long-standing emotional consequences. Adolescents who are openly gay or who are merely suspected of being so are often bullied in schools (Savin-Williams 1994). There may be links between such harassment and the worrying levels of suicide and attempted suicide among gay youth (Muehrer 1995). There are considerable problems related to substance abuse in the gay and lesbian communities that go unrecognised. Gay people are less likely to marry and have children, and are less likely to live within a mutually supportive long-term relationship (Berger 1980). As a way of compensating for these factors, they may invest more time and effort in the work place. At the time of retirement, this *raison d'être* is lost, and individuals may face greater existential anxiety and mental illness than their straight counterparts. This may be compounded by lack of support from children and the interest in grandchildren. Gay men and women who are currently at retirement age have lived much of their lives while male homosexual behaviour was illegal in Britain and 'coming out' was far more difficult than today.

What is known about the mental health of gay men and lesbians?

Despite this history of social exclusion and disadvantage, until recently there was no systematic study in Britain of the mental health and quality of life of gay men and lesbians and their needs for appropriate mental health services. Most research on the mental health of gays and lesbians has been conducted in the United States. Although there have been large surveys, most have not included appropriate comparison groups. For example, Bradford *et al.* (1994) conducted an uncontrolled survey of 1,925 lesbians in 50 states of the USA. Recruitment was not well described, but 42 per cent of question-naires were returned. Over half the sample had had suicidal thoughts and 18 per cent had attempted suicide. Thirty-two percent had been sexually assaulted. Almost 75 per cent had received counselling at some time, usually for depression. Few were open about their sexuality with their families. Cochran and Mays surveyed 829 gay male and 603 lesbian black Amer-icans who were recruited nationally in the USA through advertising, mailing businesses patronised by black gays and known social networks. Comparisons were made with published norms for the questionnaires used. Higher levels of depression were found than expected from subjects' ethnicity or gender. A small number of studies in the United States have investigated the personal and social adaptation of older gay men (Berger 1980; Bennet and Thompson 1980; Laner 1978). However, with one excep-tion (Laner 1978), the studies were uncontrolled, and used unstandardised questionnaires and/or small, unrepresentative samples. In the one controlled study of 569 gay and straight men and women, Carlson and Steuer (1985) reported a slight negative correlation between age and depression scores using the Zung self-rating depression scale in gay men. The authors concluded that ageing did not have a negative impact on self concept.

The encounter between gay people and mental health professionals

Disclosure of sexual orientation on the part of gay men and lesbians in the mental health care context is essential for the provision of effective, sensitive and individualised care. Research suggests that anti-homosexual bias is as common an occurrence for lesbian and gay individuals making contact with health and care services as it is in wider society (see Pharr 1988; Wilton 1997, 2000). However, as Wilton (2000: 6) points out 'there are no hard and fast rules about homophobia. One of the hardest things for lesbians and gay men to live with is its unpredictability'. Rather than simply focusing on the impact of homophobia Wilton (2000) also outlines the elusive but perhaps more pervasive effect that heterosexism, or 'heteronormativity', can have on the treatment experiences of lesbians and gay men. There is evidence that many gay and lesbian people attempt to hide their gay identity while in the care of mental health services (Hellman *et al.* 1996). The London-based Project for Advice, Counselling and Education (PACE) and the charity MIND, which is seeking funding for this research, have both published evidence on difficulties gay men and lesbians experience in accessing mental health care (PACE 1998; Golding 1997). These include depreciation of their domestic circumstances, refusal to accept partners as next of kin, 'voyeurism' on the part of health staff about gay lifestyles, worries about confidentiality, and fears of having their sexuality regarded as the main 'pathology' requiring discussion. In the PACE report it was claimed that:

> Judgement is made on the basis of their sexual identity and their identity as service users. Not only that, they are also discriminated against from within lesbian, gay and bisexual communities, again on the basis of their use of mental health services (PACE, 1997: 117).

While mental health professionals in the UK no longer pathologise homosexuality, many professionals are reported to display at worst overtly homophobic attitudes and at best insensitivity to sexual minorities. In response, a lesbian, gay and bisexual (LGB) affirmative strand of mental health services provision is slowly developing (Davis and Neal 1996). Mental health professionals are increasingly interested in the varying strategies used by LGB individuals to cope with social hostility and the different outcomes of these strategies in terms of self esteem and well being. However, this is a slow development and lesbian and gay users recount upsetting and disturbing encounters with mental health professionals as a result of poor training and deep-rooted mind-sets.

Gay health professionals and discrimination

Gay and lesbian health professionals themselves risk discrimination in the work place. Many are unable to be open about the gender of their partners or discuss their private lives for fear of discrimination. This has been reported over recent years in articles about the difficulties faced by gay doctors (Anonymous 1995a,b). There is also prejudice against acceptance of gays and lesbians as trainees in psychoanalysis. The traditional training institutes for psychoanalysis are known to discriminate against openly gay and lesbian applicants on the grounds that homosexuality is a mental pathology (Friedman and Lilling 1996; Bartlett *et al.* 2001).

Gay people's accounts of their experiences in mental health services

In light of recent research in Britain which shows that lesbians, gay men and bisexuals are more likely to see mental health professionals than their heterosexual counterparts (King *et al.* 2003), this chapter critically examines the nature of these encounters and the problems faced by LGB users in the mental health system. We present findings from 23 in-depth interviews with LGB individuals who were mental health service users. They recount negative experiences with clinicians as a result of poor training, lack of empathy and deep-rooted mind-sets. In particular it is shown that professionals need to strike a balance between the extremes of regarding same-sex attraction as the underlying cause of psychological difficulties, ignoring sexuality altogether and displaying excessive curiosity about how LGB people live.

Data collection

Twenty-three face-to-face interviews were conducted with individuals, nine of whom were gay men and fourteen were lesbians, who had previous experiences with mental health practitioners. The participants constituted an opportunity sample having previously taken part in a nation-wide quantitative study examining psychological well-being among gay men, lesbian and bisexuals in England and Wales (King *et al.* 2003). The three inclusion criteria for the qualitative study were that participants were over 16 years old, identified as lesbian or gay and had received treatment for a mental health issue.

The participants were recruited from a wide age range (17–64 years old) and came from all over England and Wales. They had a diverse range of experiences which included voluntary, statutory and private services (for example, residential care in psychiatric hospitals, out-patient psychiatry and psychology, long-term psychotherapy, user groups, GP services, group therapy, and counselling and therapy).

The interviews were conducted at a mutually agreed venue, took 45–60 minutes, were tape-recorded and subsequently transcribed. Written, informed consent was obtained in all cases and each participant received £20 to offset costs for taking part. The software package NVivo was used to assist with the data analysis. The authors were involved in a number of discussions about emerging themes and atypical cases.

Positive encounters

It is important to note at the outset that the intention of material in this section is to outline some of the issues and difficulties that arise in encounters between gay and lesbian people and their mental health professionals and how these impacted on the identity of being gay. We also focus on how our participants thought these difficulties might be overcome. It must be emphasised that not all informants who pointed out particular difficulties with their mental health professional found their whole experience to be negative but rather the negative experience coloured their memory of it. Indeed a number of respondents were able to recount positive encounters with mental health professionals:

> My psychologist encouraged me not to worry about being gay. He said that there was no link between me being depressed and me being gay. He was very encouraging, encouraging me not to be depressed. He was very supportive.
>
> (Male in his 40s).

> My psychologist is very helpful. He is a nice man actually ... If I ever get really bad I can pop in and get to see him ... I can go to him any time I need help. He's pleased I don't have as many panic attacks as I used to but we still have to work on going out ...
>
> (Male in his 30s).

> I am open to people who are health professionals because I think they need to know because there are health effects that sexuality confers. For example, I had to explain to my doctor that the fact [my girlfriend] had thrush meant that I needed treating for thrush as well. He obviously hadn't treated lesbians before and it hadn't twigged that [thrush] might be a problem for me too. So I had to explain that to him and once he realised he was fine.
>
> (Female in her 30s).

Among some older participants there was a common perception that, regardless of the potential shortcomings of the current service, things had improved with regard to revealing and discussing one's sexuality with mental health practitioners. The respondent quoted below, a female in her 50s who suffered sexual abuse in her teens and subsequently from depression throughout her life, reported that she felt that revealing one's sexuality is no longer as problematic as it once was:

> I have only come out recently. Had I been going through all that decision-making when I was in my teens, I would certainly have met … opposition. Certainly those doctors wouldn't have been as tolerant and understanding, those doctors through all my teenage years … They wouldn't have been as sympathetic.
>
> (Female in her 30s).

Vignette 1

Judith, 58, London.

Judith first became aware of sexual feeling towards other women around the age of eleven.

> I absolutely fell head over heals with this prefect when I was in first year, She was probably lower sixth at the time, I was 11 and she was 17. She was the antithesis of everything I knew, frightfully posh, very tall with fair curly hair and blue eyes. She was anally retentive I would say but I thought she was just an angel.

It wasn't until her 40s that she first identified with being a lesbian.

> It wasn't until my 40s that I realised that I had never stopped having crushes on women and it was only then that all the pieces of the jigsaw fitted. I can remember day-dreaming before of kissing women passionately but not really understanding that it is necessarily a sexual thing. It sounds terribly naïve doesn't it?

Coming out was a slow process.

> I would now call myself a lesbian. I had been married to a guy for 28 years who was nice but I was never attracted to him sexually, which was okay because he had a fairly low sex drive. I stopped fancying him very quickly after we got married.

Judith first suffered from depression in her 40s.

> I've had two major sessions of depression. One was the one where I remembered about being sexually abused. One was after when I came out at work and had been bullied. I was very depressed then because I

felt that I had given up on myself. Looking back too I was probably depressed in my late teens because I can remember being put on Valium. It relieved me of all my inhibitions. I remember saying something tactless to one of my teachers at school and being really shocked at myself.

She found many of the mental health professionals she encountered to be empathetic around her sexuality.

Mental health professionals were okay. My GP was great because I had realised a bit before that that I thought I was a lesbian and I think it probably put a few cracks in my psyche. I told my GP about my feeling and said that I feel such a fool. But she told me that it was not that unusual. So my GP was okay and never stopped treating me like a normal person. I had a really good counsellor. On one occasion I even took my husband and we discussed our marriage. She was incredibly helpful and it was great to have somebody who you felt you could be really open to. Quite often I would project things on to counsellors which they were not thinking at all. No, they were not judgemental. Most of them understood perfectly what I was talking about.

Homophobia and heterosexism

In his studies of attitudes toward homosexuality among counsellors, Rudolph (1989, 1990) pointed out that many therapists may not be aware of their unconscious anti-LGB attitudes that could contribute to inconsistent therapeutic positions and actions with their LGB patients. He reported that the attitudes of professional counsellors toward sexuality were often ambiguous. In many cases individual counsellors contended that LGB people were capable of functioning in any given context and yet their sexual orientation hindered their performance in certain situations.

Studies of behaviour therapists (Davison and Wilson 1974) and psychoanalysts (Lilling and Friedman 1995; Bartlett *et al.* 2001) have shown that most rejected a pathological model of homosexuality and felt that having a LGB sexual orientation was not of itself an impediment to quality of life and psychological well-being. Few mental health practitioners have been specifically trained, however, to surmount the anti-LGB bias which they share with wider society (Sayce 1995), and indeed there are those employed in the mental health services who have been trained to regard non-heterosexual sexualities as mental disorders. While certainly not the norm, a number of respondents in the study cited examples of overtly homophobic experiences in their encounters with mental health services. Below is the testimony of a 35-year-old woman who was undergoing treatment for manic depression at a London hospital:

> I went to see a psychiatric nurse who was assessing me. She was com-
> pletely homophobic . . . she was so rude to me and so horrible to me . . .
> and I was very, very vulnerable and I thought I just can't face it. She just
> completely rejected me and said 'well do you think that being in a
> lesbian relationship is going to help you through all this?' She said
> the most unbelievable stuff. I just terminated.
>
> (Female in her 30s).

A man in his 30s on medication for depression and stress described the
process of actually being asked to leave his GP practice, a reason that he
clearly attributed to his sexual orientation:

> I asked my GP for a hepatitis injection. He asked me why I wanted it
> and I said I was gay apart from everything else. He just looked at me
> and three days later I got a letter saying I could find another GP.
>
> (Male in his 20s).

Whilst we do not want to downplay the effects of such homophobic
responses this was not the most dominant criticism emerging from the personal narratives of the participants in the study. Explicit negativity from
practitioners seemed to be the exception rather than the rule. Instead, the
majority of the respondents described experiences that involved far more
subtle forms of discrimination, which were underpinned by an almost universal assumption of heterosexuality. Heterosexism assumes the supremacy
of social practice, cultural structures and idioms related to heterosexuality.
According to the Group for the Advancement of Psychiatry (2000) this
conviction is 'usually accompanied by a therapist's denial and devaluation
of vital aspects of lesbian or gay emotional growth and ignores the development of healthy interpersonal relationships' (2000:28). Heterosexist
encounters are related in the quotations below:

> What I found really hard about the mental health services when I think
> about it now in retrospect is that sexuality is completely ignored unless
> you're heterosexual and I think to say that it's completely assumed that
> everyone is heterosexual unless you particularly state otherwise. They
> never ever, they don't seem to be able to see this point and I've put it to
> them a lot of times. People think they are politically correct and equal
> opportunity and they say they have no problem with gay women but if
> you really look at the way they practice and how much they take for
> granted that you're straight immediately makes it quite hard. It means
> you have to come out deliberately with your sexuality whereas hetero-
> sexual people don't have to say 'I am a heterosexual'.
>
> (Female in her 30s).

I often raised the issue about sexuality and how it was ignored and I think it runs through the service ... it's not necessarily deliberate or overt, people don't even know they are doing it but the fact that they assume you've got a boyfriend or might be looking for a boyfriend if you're a woman, there's this assumption all the time.

(Female in her 20s).

People could be trained to have an awareness to start with that the client in front of them may or may not be completely heterosexual, they could be anything sexually. They will assume you're straight.

(Male in his 40s).

As well as a presumption of heterosexuality, there were also accounts of mental health practitioners' unwillingness to draw out or engage with the issues surrounding their clients' sexuality. In the wider world 'lesbians and gay men must constantly decide whether or not it is safe to "come out", what the likely consequences will be and whether or not they can trust the judgement of the other people involved' (Wilton 2002). Participants in the present study made links between the professional showing a sense that he or she was aware of LGB issues to their own sense of safety in discussing aspects of their sexuality. Many however, felt that they were unable to express themselves properly, as recounted by a Manchester man in his 40s:

I had never said I was gay before to anybody properly. I really wanted to and hoped that it would help me with [my depression]. I was very disappointed that my psychiatrist didn't want to know and didn't help me talk through it ... he seemed to just change the subject and [talk about] something else.

(Male in his 40s).

Another participant had received a variety of services for long-term depression over the course of seven years, exacerbated by her father's rejection of her because of her sexuality. She described her difficulties in raising the issue of sexuality with her professionals and her confusion about her sexual orientation at the age of fourteen:

I don't think that [mental health practitioners] ever raised [sexuality], they never pushed it ... they certainly never pursued it or helped me pursue it. If I ever did talk about it, it would have been very general, they certainly wouldn't have given me enough room to explore It ... I think a lot of my problems emotionally ... were connected to my sexuality and my suppression of that and my feelings that I had to suppress it.

(Female in her 20s).

Vignette 2

Sheila, 36 years old, Bristol.
  Sheila first became aware that she was a lesbian in her mid-20s.

> That is when I became aware of issues of being gay and gradually
> coming to terms with it. It wasn't something I particularly wanted to
> be or anything. Then I looked back on my life in a different way and
> identified feelings I had when that happened when I was much younger,
> even a child or teenager. Now I think they are what would be called
> sexual feelings. I never identified them as that.

She was surprised by her first crush.

> It was quite sudden, someone who did become a friend and she actually
> made advances towards me ... I got into a relationship with her. I
> would always call myself gay. I've never liked the word lesbian.

Coming out was a slow process.

> Probably it has taken me several years to feel okay about being com-
> pletely open with most people except my family. I've never been overly
> open with any single member of my family. My current partner is
> accepted as part of the family but it's not actually spoken about, not
> actually given a word even though it is patently obvious.

Sheila has never much enjoyed the gay scene.

> It's alright but my early experiences were at women-only discos. It is
> quite a shallow world I think. Although just a year ago I went to
> Blackpool and deliberately went to a gay place which was really good
> fun. But I think the fact that the gay scene revolves around nightclubs
> and music and drinking and that experience is a shallow experience
> for me.

Sheila first suffered from depression around the age of 10.

> I was really young and I knew it was a different feeling than I had
> before. I distinctly remember actually when I felt depression, it was
> physical but I remember the feeling, it was absolutely horrible. I remem-
> ber trying to describe it to my mother but she didn't say anything of any
> use or any help. I suffered from depression right through my teens. I
> think it important to say that I think the depression was for a reason, it
> didn't just come over me for no reason. I know that there were reasons

why I got depressed as a little kid, the predominant one being that my father was an alcoholic. There were so many things going on at home that I found difficult. I wanted to hide it and went out of my way to appear happy.

When she was 19 she suffered a breakdown.

I had just moved to Bristol and had a boyfriend I thought I was in love with. It is a bit vague but I suddenly started becoming psychotic and paranoid. I started reading the Bible and was thinking it was written in code and was terribly complicated. It just got worse and worse and I got madder and madder.

Her parents had her sectioned.

I got taken away in an ambulance. I agreed to go but I thought it was my parents just playing a joke that had gone wrong. I definitely thought I wasn't mad and I thought that when I got away from my parents everyone would realise that I wasn't mad. My first memory was of a dingy ward with come peculiar people. I couldn't work out how I had gone from an ordinary life to being locked up somewhere so strange. I just hadn't realised what psychiatric hospitals are actually like. It was crap. Her first stay was three months. I stayed five days a week and was allowed home to my parents at weekends. I was given a whole range of drugs. I don't know what any of them were. I was given ECT completely against my will. But the main treatment was drugs, every day. On the second night I was sexually abused by one of the staff, a man. That obviously made the whole experience very traumatic and there was nobody I could tell. The place felt like a prison, there were bars on the windows of my room. My abuser abused other patients as well and it was very frightening because of the manner in which he would do things and the secrecy around it. He was very conniving.

Sheila became an outpatient for two years.

But after two years from my first stay at the hospital I became psychotic again and was sectioned again. Everyday was indescribably boring. I was young and energetic and was used to doing lots of things. They kept changing my diagnosis all the time. First they said I was schizophrenic, one said it was toxic psychosis, another that it was hypomania. Then they said after a while it was just depression. I saw a psychiatrist regularly.

She noted the presumption of heterosexuality among the mental health professionals.

What I found really hard about the mental health services was that sexuality is really completely ignored. They all think you are heterosexual. You would have to tell them you are gay. They are certainly not going to ask you. They never seem to be able to see this point and I have put it to them a lot of times. People think they are basically correct and all into equal opportunities and they say they have no problem with gay women but when you look at the way they practice and how much they take for granted that you're straight, it makes it quite hard. It means that you have to deliberately come out with your sexuality whereas heterosexual people don't have to say: I am a heterosexual.

She remembers one particular incident when she discussed her sexuality.

I remember one time I mentioned to a psychiatrist that I was a lesbian. I had just started a relationship and I wanted her to say it was okay. She did say it was okay but very much thought that it was just a phase. She said that she had a very strong attachment to a woman when she was younger but that she had got over it and was now married. So I thought for a while that it was nice of her to be that open with me. It made me feel a little better that she didn't treat me any worse. But she wasn't taking me seriously and really wanted to reassure me that it was a phase and that I would grow out of it.

Looking back Sheila thinks her treatment for mental health problems could have benefited from more attention to her sexuality.

I think that sexuality is a very important issue. I wouldn't have said that ten years ago when I was sectioned but then that's what I really needed help with. A holistic approach to look at my whole life which would have included sexuality, regardless of what that sexuality is.

Misattribution and stereotypes

Participants who did discuss their sexuality reported that they often received not necessarily negative, but clumsy and ill-informed responses. As reported in a previous study (King *et al.* 2003), 18 per cent of gay men, 18 per cent of lesbians, 33 per cent of bisexual men and 13 per cent of bisexual women who had seen a mental health professional for emotional difficulties stated that they had been told that their sexuality was the root of their problems. While in some cases this may be true, in many cases, rather than providing a safe, affirmative environment for their gay and lesbian clients, these kinds of assertions assumed that sexuality was a problem for the client. It may well be that practitioners lack a repertoire of questions about social and sexual history appropriate to LGB people or are unaware of why they might be necessary. However, when the mental health professional places too much emphasis on sexuality or regards it as central to the client relationship, this is also problematic. This issue is illustrated by the two accounts presented below:

> *Interviewer*: Can you describe a time when a mental health professional implied that your sexual orientation might be the reason why you felt depressed or anxious?

> *Respondent*: I did get told that I was trying to live two lives, that it was the sexuality that was causing the problem ... What they also said was that being brought up in Dr Barnardos, because I've always been brought up in a male environment and never mixed with females, they thought it was because I didn't know the other gender.
>
> (Male in his 20s).

> *Interviewer*: Has anyone suggested that your sexual orientation might be related to your mental health problems?

> *Respondent*: My psychiatrist brought up [the subject of my sexual orientation] during one of our meetings. He annoyed me actually because he turned round and said 'do you think you need counselling sessions with a specialist counsellor?'. I said 'what do you mean by a specialist counsellor?' Well he said 'somebody of your gender'. I said that it doesn't matter if it's male or female. He said 'I mean your sexuality'.
>
> (Female in her 30s).

In other cases, participants related how their mental health professionals focused on sexual orientation as a therapeutic issue when it was not essential to the concerns that brought them into therapy.

> I don't like talking to my psychiatrist [about my sexual orientation] because I don't see it as an issue that needs to be aired or anything. I'd rather get to the root of why I'm like I am and not put anything else on to think well maybe that's the cause of it. But he kept insisting on talking about.
>
> (Male in his 40s).

The following participant, having been previously diagnosed as suffering from a personality disorder, reported that he had yet to trust a psychiatrist enough to discuss his sexuality for fear that he would be judged negatively for being gay and that his sexuality would be implicated as a cause of his mental health problems. It is instructive that in his many years of treatment for his mental health the 'opportunity has not arisen' for him to discuss his sexuality and that he 'would love to be able to talk to them' about it.

> I have the fear that I will be judged in a way that they would take the sexuality side and take it as the problem rather than what is the problem which I don't think is the sexual part of me. If I wasn't gay I'd still have the same problems but I always felt that if I talked about my sexuality to professionals I'd be uncomfortable ... Unless I met somebody different who I would feel at ease with I haven't met them yet that I could do that with.
>
> (Male in his 50s).

Defensive language of clients

A number of participants, who reported positive experiences of coming out in a mental health setting, used language which revealed their low expectations of the outcome and how they had anticipated negative reactions from their practitioner. In the examples presented below the GPs were 'not judgemental at all' and 'not nasty or unpleasant' and the social worker 'didn't have a problem with it' when each of the participants revealed his or her sexuality. This perhaps indicates how many LGB people have been socialised to be defensive and to expect negative reactions when declaring their sexual orientation to others in the wider social context. So when the response is positive as in each of the examples cited, the double negative language reflects the internalised expectation of rejection or disapproval:

> My GP works as a doctor in the gay village, so it's gay friendly. I find that quite helpful because if you have any issues, they're not judgemental at all.
>
> (Male in his 40s).

> My social worker was ... pretty good actually. Obviously she'd read in my file that I was gay and she didn't have a problem with it, whereas some of the other professionals would turn up their noses at it.
>
> (Male in his 30s).

> I'm open to people who are health professionals because I think they need to know because there are health effects which sexuality confers ... [My GP] was not nasty or unpleasant at all and he's one of the few men I've ever come to trust ... I worry about seeing anyone different.
>
> (Female in her 30s).

Perhaps not surprisingly, those participants in the study who had had encounters with LGB practitioners found their potential empathy an advantage. They suggested that LGB therapists and clinicians were more likely to have an awareness of the needs of their LGB clients than their heterosexual counterparts.

> I know some lesbians who don't care and are not interested in the sexuality of their psychiatrist. But I thought ... if she was a lesbian she might be more empathetic, they'd understand some of the issues, they'd have been through coming out and all the rest of it.
>
> (Female in her 30s).

> I think seeing a counsellor who is gay makes a difference as well, because even the best of person-centred counsellors there could still be some homophobia [and] as much as they might try [to cover it up] it would show.
>
> (Male in his 30s).

> [The counsellor] said 'well I'm in a lesbian relationship. I've been in one for the last five years ...' It was such a relief. The millstone I had put round my neck about how difficult and impossible this was going to be, just fell off ... because there was someone else who knew and who had tried to be normal and discovered that she wasn't normal in that sense and was happily living in a lesbian relationship.
>
> (Female in her 30s).

Of course, those lesbian and gay clients, when confronted with an uneasy interaction or situation with a practitioner, may have insufficient presence of mind or self-confidence to assert themselves in such circumstances. They may feel unable to change the conduct of the practitioner, resolve an uncomfortable situation, or speak openly about their discomfort. For a vulnerable client, this may stem from a history of discrimination, a power imbalance in the client/practitioners relationship, and/or past memories of difficult experiences. The two accounts below reflect this vulnerability:

> *Interviewer*: How would you describe your relationship with your psychiatrist?

> *Respondent*: I wouldn't even call it a relationship ... I felt like this object he was going to fix. I didn't feel like a person at all. He used to just sit there and peer at me. He was very cold and distant. I didn't know what to do, how to change [the situation]. I didn't really want to talk about anything at all with the psychiatrist.
>
> (Female in her 40s).

I have never felt comfortable with [my psychiatrist] when it comes to sexuality. I feel stupid and powerless and never really say the right thing. That's a confidence thing. If I had the confidence I would say 'no I don't agree with you'. But I just become passive and let him do the talking even though I don't agree with him.

(Male in his 30s).

Vignette 3

John, 36, London

John first became aware of being attracted to members of the same sex when he was in his mid-teens.

I suppose I was 15 or 16. It's very confusing. I get attracted to women and I get attracted to men. I would say I get attracted to men more than I get attracted to women but if I go out with a man it's the actual sex I can't handle. I find it hard because all my friends are straight whereas I am I suppose bisexual. I have some gay friends but some of them don't know my sexuality. I find it all very difficult about who to tell. Because all my friends are straight then sometimes I don't want to be gay.

He is not out to any of his family or at work.

I haven't discussed it and I never will. They don't need to know, they wouldn't feel happier or less happy so there's no point. They don't live in the area so they are not around all the time. But even if they did live close to me I would still be unlikely to tell them as I don't want to.

He found the gay scene a positive experience.

I love it because I can be myself. I have gone through the sex stage where you have to have sex and all that. It's just weird, everyone's just at ease and just being themselves and I can be myself and I find that really, really brilliant.

Mental health problems first emerged in his late teens.

I first became mentally ill when I was 17 or 18. I have been clinically depressed. I do have general feelings of depression most of the time. I'm an outgoing person so I hide it quite well. I also feel anxious a lot of the time, I get very anxious when I go out. I can start to get panic attacks and go off a bit. I was sent to see a psychiatrist first when I was 17. I had to go into hospital for a year which dealt with personality disorders. That was very intensive therapy and I was never going to go back, it was awful, I would never want to go there. So in the last 15 years I have been involved with psychiatrists or hospitals or social workers. The majority of psychiatrists I have hated particularly when I was really down. When I started to get better I liked them a bit more.

He has never discussed his sexuality with a professional.

I never have in all these years. I fear that I will be judged in a way that would take the sexuality side of it and take it as the problem rather than what is the problem that I don't feel is the sexual part of me. If I wasn't gay I'd still have the same problems but I have always felt that if I talked about my sexuality to professionals I'd be uncomfortable and would not be able to justify how I felt. Unless I met somebody different who I would feel at ease with, I haven't met them yet that I could do that with. I don't think they would treat me the same way. I would have loved to have talked about my sexuality on a number of occasions but the opportunity hasn't arisen and the right person has not been available to do that with. And they have never come out and asked me if I was gay or if I have a sexual problem so I have never had to explain anything away.

Conclusions

The process by which gay men and lesbians have achieved a coherent sense of identity over the past century has been affected by deeply held views in society that homosexuality is a mental disorder. This has made the shaping of homosexual identities much more complex than in other groups such as ethnic minorities or the disabled. When parents reject their gay or lesbian children, it means that discrimination has reached into the heart of the nuclear family and torn it apart, something rarely seen in other settings. Thus, when mental health problems do occur in gay and lesbian people, feelings of shame and exposure that are almost inevitable in adolescence may be re-awakened and pose a threat to their sense of identity. Although anti-homosexual bias in mental health services is diminishing in Britain, significant problems still exist. One of the common themes across many of the disparate clinical encounters presented in this chapter is the lack of empathy on the part of many clinicians and their lack of understanding of gay and lesbian identities. Disclosure of sexual orientation on the part of gay and lesbian individuals in the mental health care context is essential for the provision of effective, sensitive and individualised care. Failure to establish rapport and communication between practitioners and clients is linked to lower rates of satisfaction and often ends in disengagement or drop-out (Tantum 2002). The instances of failure stem from simple ignorance about human sexuality and sexual orientation and lesbian and gay development throughout the life cycle, and the sense of identity in gay and lesbian communities. Education and training can tackle this kind of lack of experience and knowledge. However, inadequate empathy on the part of a professional might be a symptom with complex psychological, social and cultural roots. While therapeutic empathy is a valuable approach, it is limited. According to a publication by the Group for the Advancement of Psychiatry (2000), psychotherapists are akin to 'those social anthropologists who achieve the goal of exploring unfamiliar ways of life sensitively and cautiously, remaining aware of differences but not assigning value judgements from their own culture to the culture under study' (2000:29). The Group argues that much like social scientists, mental health professionals need to comprehend how beliefs and practices and outlook that may seem unfamiliar and alienating to them can be coherent and natural to others.

Acknowledgements

We wish to acknowledge with gratitude all those who made the research study possible: The Community Fund for funding the study, Mind, the National Association for Mental Health for their crucial input at all stages of the research, the participants who took part in the face-to-face interviews, and other members of the study team including Katherine Johnson, Angus Ramsay, Clive Cort, James Warner and Oliver Davidson.

References

Anonymous (1995a) 'Being a gay doctor', *Student British Medical Journal*, 3:385–6.
Anonymous (1995b) 'Being a gay medical student', *Student British Medical Journal*, 3:386.
Bartlett A., King M. and Phillips P. (2001) 'Straight talking – an investigation of the attitudes and practice of psychoanalysts and psychotherapists in relation to gays and lesbians', *British Journal of Psychiatry*, 179:545–9.
Bennett K.C. and Thompson N.L. (1980) 'Social and Psychological functioning of the ageing male homosexual', *British Journal of Psychiatry*, 137:361–370.
Berger R.M. (1980) 'Psychological adaptation of the older homosexual male', *Journal of Homosexuality*, 5:161–75.
Bewley S. (1997) 'Medical students: a survey of deans of medical schools', paper presented to the conference, *Gay and Lesbian Mental Health* at the Royal Society of Medicine, London, 14 October.
Bhugra D. and King M.B. (1989) 'Controlled comparison of attitudes of psychiatrists, general practitioners, homosexual doctors and homosexual men to male homosexuality', *Journal of The Royal Society of Medicine*, 82:603–5.
Bradford J., Ryan C. and Rothblum E.D. (1994) 'National lesbian health care survey: implications for mental health care', *Journal of Clinical and Consulting Psychology*; 62:228–42.

Cabaj R. and Stein T.S. (eds) (1996) *Textbook of Homosexuality and Mental Health*, Washington, American Psychiatric Press.

Carlson H.M. and Steuer J. (1985) 'Age, sex-role categorisation and psychological health in American homosexual and heterosexual men and women', *Journal of Social Psychology*, 125:203–11.

Davies D. and Neal C. (eds) (1996) *Pink Therapy: A Guide for Counsellors and Therapists Working with Lesbian, Gay and Bisexual Clients*, Buckingham, Open University Press.

Davison G.C. and Wilson G.T. (1974) 'Goals and strategies in behavioural treatment of homosexual pedophilia: comments on a case study', *Journal of Abnormal Psychology*, 83, 196–8.

Drescher J. (1998) 'I'm your handyman. A history of reparative therapies', *Journal of Homosexuality*, 36:19–42.

Evans J.K., Bingham J.S., Pratt K. and Carne C.A. (1993) 'Attitudes of medical students to HIV and AIDS', *Genitourinary Medicine*, 69:377–80.

Friedman R.C. and Lilling A.A. 'An empirical study of the beliefs of psychoanalysts about scientific and clinical dimensions of male homosexuality', *Journal Homosexuality* 32:79–89.

Greene B. (1994) 'Ethnic-minority lesbians and gay men: mental health and treatment issues', *Journal of Clinical and Consulting Psychology*, 62:243–51.

Group for the Advancement of Psychiatry (2000) *Homosexuality and the Mental Health Professions: The Impact of Bias*, Hillsdale, NJ, The Analytic Press.

Haldeman D.C. (1994) 'The practice and ethics of sexual orientation conversion therapy', *Journal of Clinical and Consulting Psychology*, 62:221–7.

Hellman R.E., Stanton M., Lee J., Tytun A., Vachon R. 'Treatment of homosexual alcoholics in government-funded agencies: provider training and attitudes', *Hospital and Community Psychiatry* 40:1163–1168, 1989.

Johnson A.M., Mercer C.H., Erens B. *et al.* (2001) 'Sexual behaviour in Britain: partnerships, practices and HIV risk behaviours', *Lancet*, 358, 1835–42.

King M.B. and Bartlett A. (1999) 'British psychiatry and homosexuality', *British Journal of Psychiatry*, 174:106–13.

King M. and McKeown E. (2003) *Minority Report: Mental health and Social Well Being of Gay men, Lesbians and Bisexuals in England and Wales*, London, Mind (in press).

King M., McKeown E., Warner J., Ramsay A., Johnson K., Cort C., Wright L., Blizard R. and Davidson O. (2003) 'Mental health and quality of life of gay men and lesbians in England and Wales: a controlled, cross-sectional survey', *British Journal of Psychiatry* (in press).

King M., Smith G. and Bartlett A. (2003) 'Treatments of homosexuality in Britain since the 1950s. Paper II – The experience of professionals', *British Medical Journal* (in press).

Laner M.R. (1978) 'Growing older male: heterosexual and homosexual', *The Gerontologist*, 18:496–501.

Lilling A. and Friedman R.C. (1995) 'Bias towards gay patients by psychoanalytic clinicians: an empirical investigation', *Archives of Sexual Behaviour*, 24, 563–70.

Muehrer P. (1995) 'Suicide and sexual orientation: a critical summary of recent research and directions for future research', *Suicide and Life-Threatening Behavior*, 25 (suppl):72–81.

McColl P. (1994) 'Homosexuality and mental health services', *British Medical Journal* 308:550–1.

PACE (Project for Advice, Counselling and Education) (1998) *Diagnosis: Homophobic. The Experiences of Lesbians, Gay Men and Bisexuals in Mental Health Services*, London, PACE.

PACE (Project for Advice Counselling and Education) (1998) *Diagnosis: Homophobic. The experiences of lesbians, gay men and bisexuals in mental health services*, London, PACE.

Pharr S. (1988) *Homophobia: a weapon of sexism*, Inverness, CA, Chardon Press.

Rogers A. (1998) *BMA News Review*, May, 27.

Rudolph, J. (1989) 'Counsellors' attitudes toward homosexuality: some tentative findings', *Psychological Reports*, 66:1352–4.

Rudolph J. (1989) 'Effects of affirmative gay psychology workshop on counsellors' authoritarianism', *Psychological Reports*, 65, 945–6.

Savin-Williams R.C. (1994) 'Verbal and physical abuse as stressors in the lives of lesbian, gay male, and bisexual youths: associations with school problems, running away, substance abuse, prostitution, and suicide', *Journal of Clinical and Consulting Psychology*, 62:261–9.

Sayce L. (1995) *Breaking the link between homosexuality and mental illness*, London, Mind.

Sell R.L., Wells J.A. and Wypij D. (1995) 'The prevalence of homosexual behaviour and attraction in the United States, the United Kingdom and France: results of national population-based samples', *Archives of Sexual Behaviour*, 24: 235–48.

Smith G., Bartlett A. and King M. (2003) 'Treatments of homosexuality in Britain since the 1950s. Paper I – The experience of patients', *British Medical Journal*, (in press).

Wilton T. (1997) *Good For You: A Handbook to Lesbian Health and Wellbeing*, London, Continuum International Publishing Group.

Wilton T. (2000) 'Sexualities' in *Health and Social Care: A Textbook*, Buckingham, Open University Press.

9

Life narratives, health and identity

Mildred Blaxter

Introduction

Much of what we believe we know about identity and health derives from life narratives. Data may range from responses to semi-structured research questions to long 'literary' biographical accounts, and from brief stories of health-related incidents to whole life histories, but always they are not just stories but vehicles for making sense of a life. Through narrative, people rearrange their experience, present their actions for judgement, and come to articulate their situation in the social world. Indeed, identity *is* a life story: an 'internalised integration of past, present and anticipated future' (McAdams 1989: 161). They are also a demonstration of the broader cultural world within which identity has a place, perhaps invoking prototypical worlds in which events unfold and actions occur in an understandable way (Garro 1994). Narratives force a revision of histories and identities, and describe how the self undergoes change within some basic continuity.

This is specially true of narratives of chronic illness, which presents particular and probably permanent challenges to identity. As Radley (1993) noted, illness becomes a context or frame within which the rest of life can be evaluated; it precipitates crises of identity, and requires negotiation of who one is with family, friends and society in general. As Bury (2001: 267) pointed out, special interest in lay narratives arose in part because of the growing impact in modern times of degenerative and chronic illness, where 'the contingencies of everyday life assert themselves, and the subjective patient view becomes audible once more'. Frank, in the classic book *The Wounded Storyteller* (1995), had similarly argued that as acute illness gives way to chronic, individuals need to make sense of their experience and 'tell their stories'.

This chapter uses some original data, set in the context of many other studies, to demonstrate these interactive processes. Identity is shown as a grid through which health and illness are perceived and given meaning, and in turn health and illness construct identity, both framed within given cultural parameters of, for instance, gender, class, and social history.

Particularly, attention will be paid to the form, structure, story-telling conventions, and purpose of narrative accounts.

The heyday of the illness narrative in the literature of sociology and social psychology was perhaps the 1980s and earlier 1990s. Many of the classic studies date from that period. The topic may be less popular now, and, speculatively, this may be related to the theory of post-modern identity, seen as increasingly fluid, multiple, dissolved, and lacking in continuity and structure. Such deconstruction of the self 'leaves identities floating on a realm of fleeting moments, transitory encounters, eternal presents' (Elliott 2001: 146).

In this light the concept of an 'identity' revealed or expressed in a life story (even at one moment and contingent on the purpose of one occasion) may be held to present problems, but one of the objectives of this chapter is, in fact, to explore whether people do indeed still construct life-long identities around health and illness experience.

Narrative genres

Various types of narrative genre have been identified in the literature, though none seems adequate to summarise the whole range of possible forms of narrative. A health narrative is a *story*, whether told logically and continuously or in fragmented parts which go back and forth: a story with a plot. Frank (1995), examining published illness narratives to understand the cumulative changes in the self found there, distinguished three basic plots:

- restitution, or the effort towards the cure and restoration of the self;
- quest, or self-transformation into a new self;
- chaos, describing a life that cannot get better.

Denzin (1986), also basing the analysis on written life histories, similarly distinguished three basic macrostructures:

- stable narratives, recounted in real time as if they were clinical case-histories;
- progressive personal narratives, reconstructions in terms of personal goals, which can be what Denzin calls 'one person clinical trials', or personal detective stories;
- regressive narratives, similarly personal reconstructions, but in the form of tragedies.

Bury (2001) discussing narratives of chronic illness, also suggested three types:

- contingent narratives, about the origins of a disease, its causes, and its immediate effects on daily life;
- moral narratives, which account for changes in the illness, the person, and the resultant social identity, and re-establish moral status;
- core narratives, which make connections between lay experiences and deeper cultural levels of meaning.

It is commonly pointed out that core narratives can take any of the classical forms: epic or heroic, tragic, comic or ironic, didactic or romantic. While one of these can be an overriding theme (as in the epic/heroic and comic/ironic tales of ulcerative colitis sufferers in Kelly and Dickenson 1997), one narrative may include elements of several. Jordens *et al.* (2001) analysing accounts of colorectal cancer, examined 'generic complexity', or the extent to which different genres could be mixed in one narrative. Distinguishing a number of types of sub-narrative – for instance, 'anecdote', where the speaker is sharing a reaction with the audience; 'exemplum', where a moral judgement is made; or 'observation', where a personal response is being shared – these authors suggested that these are almost always mixed, and the degree of generic complexity is related to the degree of life disruption that the speaker has suffered.

Narrative purposes

It can be noted that all these are narratives of *illness*, and usually of specific disease. Whole life stories of 'normal' mixed health and illness are less common in research, and among literary narratives are less usually analysed from the point of view of health. The circumstances and purposes of narrative production – the objective of a research interview, for instance – must of course affect both form and content. What are people doing when they provide narratives? Interview narratives are different from written accounts, as they are the outcome of situated speech, coloured to a greater or lesser extent by question and answer. They are 'more fragile, inconsistent and incomplete than a self-consciously constructed text' (Kirmayer 2000). Frank (1997) suggests that literary accounts sit in between research data and *belles lettres*. They may be analysed as data – a notable example is Crossley (2003) – but their form and quality do depend on the writer's ability to express themselves. This should not be a major factor in interview data, though of course it often is. More importantly, published literary accounts are not meant to generalise. As Frank notes, they may appeal to the experience of others who can empathise, but this illness experience is being presented and published as worth reading precisely *because* it is singular, an individual story.

Still focusing on illness, many authors have analysed the deliberate construction of narratives in therapeutic settings as an interactive process. Del

Vecchio Good *et al.* (1994), for instance, considered the concept of 'therapeutic emplotment', the way in which a plot is negotiated within clinical time by patients and clinicians. In emplotting cancer narratives, therapists deliberately control both hope and despair. Mattingly (1994) similarly discusses how therapists actively struggle to shape events into a coherent whole for stroke patients. Brody (1994) and King and Stanford (1992) are other examples of narrative as a doctor's tool.

The narratives of people's own perceptions and experiences of illness, especially chronic disease, often have the overt purpose for both researchers and subjects of being 'useful' (helping clinicians or others to understand). For instance, a patient with severe liver disease said:

> If there's anything I know, or anything I've done, anything at all, that's going to help someone else, I'm delighted. It's something that I can do that.
>
> (Blaxter and Cyster 1984).

In the genre described earlier as 'quests', narratives very often have a regenerative nature, and are explicitly part of the search for a new identity, embracing, incorporating, resisting or rejecting the disease. Normalising and minimising narratives have the purpose of 'allowing feelings of being different from others to be pushed backstage' (Kelleher 1988). Hawkins (1990) suggested that in their regenerative nature chronic illness accounts may be replacing the established genre of stories of religious conversion. Kleinman (1988) defined narrative broadly as the form in which patients shape and give voice to their suffering, and notes that the emphasis on suffering may derive from the medical interests.

Of course different forms of suffering, different parts of the body which are affected, may mean different effects on identity. The particularity of disease is well expressed by a sufferer from macular degeneration:

> It was as if my I had been displaced and now reached out to you from the vantage part of my Eye – *one* particular part of my body.
>
> (Wikan 2000: 222).

Similarly, other sufferers from particular conditions may stress special effects upon their identity: rheumatoid arthritis and issues of control, autonomy and coping (Williams 1993); multiple sclerosis and attitudes of mind, particularly in contested diagnoses (Pollock 1993); HIV and strategies of social change (Carricaburu and Pierret 1995); cancers and gender identity (Hunt 2000); and very many others. Thus the *topic* of the narrative – the specific disease – has to be taken into consideration in stories of chronic or life-threatening illness. 'Different conditions carry with them different connotations and imagery. These differences may have a profound influence on how individuals regard themselves, and how they think others see them' (Bury 1991: 453).

However, a complete life narrative is not, ordinarily, exclusively about suffering. Health is, in fact, less easy to talk about, and most data concern illness, not health. There are exceptions, where people have been selected as research subjects in some random fashion, not because they belong to a diagnostic group or are in contact with health services, but rather are 'ordinary' people with varied health experiences (Herzlich 1973; Backett 1992; Pierret 1993). Even in these samples, however, more general discussion of health experiences often tends to turn to narratives of illness. Moreover, special groups – notably the socially disadvantaged, whose health is likely to be poor – are commonly chosen for obvious reasons of policy interest (Blaxter and Paterson 1982; Cornwell 1984). The health histories of those who see themselves as essentially healthy are rare.

The context and purpose of the narratives cannot be ignored. Many of the studies of 'well' populations have purposes which are secondary to looking at life histories: purposes such as the study of lay concepts of health, or of attitudes to health, or of views of health services, which are likely to have health promotion or health policy objectives. If respondents see the purpose of the enquiry as connected with health education, if they believe that they are being asked to justify their health behaviour, they will of course comply with this agenda. They will focus on lifestyle and choice, responsibility and chance, the story of *why* health events happened (and to me) (Davison *et al.* 1992). As in tales of chronic illness, moral narratives are likely. The narrative has to use what is socially acceptable, credible, and morally sound.

The less structured the form of interviewing the more the data have to be built, as Garro (1994) noted, around what people themselves judge to be worth talking about. Essentially, they are attempts to convince a listener of their point of view. The story of a sickness may 'even function as a political commentary, pointing a finger of condemnation at perceived injustice and the personal experience of oppression' (Kleinman 1988: 50).

Narrative conventions: plot and story

As Riessman (1990) argued, the *how* of the telling is as important as what is said. Narrative analysis breaks down the organisation of the discourse into segments, and looks at the underlying structure and movement. The tone of the speech – its vocabulary, underlying emotion, and eager or reluctant flow – is also illuminating. Narrative is a performance, and sometimes it is overtly dramatising, with reported speech and detailed description offered as proof of 'how it was'. Sometimes there are non-narrative insertions, segments which report thoughts and actions, but have only a tenuous relationship to the 'plot'. At the other extreme, heightened speech and the use of metaphor transform illness symptoms into symbols of change, as Radley noted 'reflecting one reality through another':

> To speak of one's own illness as 'a crossroads' is not only to organise one's meaning in a particular way, but also to give all forms of crossing a symbolic value they might not have had beforehand.
>
> (Radley 1993: 113).

There are many definitions of 'narrative' and of 'story', but the position taken here is that of Good and DelVecchio Good (1994): life history interviews are composed as a corpus of shorter stories. The pattern of the history moves, as Bruner (1986) suggested, between memories – which can be transformed, sometimes even in the process of telling – and futures, continually being modified. The building blocks of narrative at the smallest level are turning-points, metaphors, remembered moments. At a larger level they are stories, self-contained episodes with a beginning, a middle and an end, and usually a 'point' or moral. Riessman (1990) suggested that stories can be distinguished from 'habitual narratives' which tell of the general course of events over time rather than one specific event. The structure can easily be seen by looking at pages of interview transcript. Some respondents are able to create a careful and logical narrative in proper time sequence and without pause. Other interviews (not usually the most successful) are merely series of brief questions and answers from beginning to end. By far the majority of interview transcripts, however, consist of some pages of question and answer interspersed with blocks, sometimes many pages long, of uninterrupted text. These are the 'stories', often told in a different style (more vivid, more emotional, with faster speech and more colourful language) to the rest of the interview. Almost always their overarching theme is of identity and its creation, change, and display, and it will be suggested that it is the analysis of these – their plot, objective, tone – which offers the clearest picture of how identity is related to health.

Data being used here

A selection of life histories is used to explore some of the points which have been discussed, applying them to the relationship of health to identity. The presentation of narrative data presents special difficulties, unless there is recourse to the single case-history (or a lengthy book): Denzin (1986) introduced the idea of the 'universal singular', the notion that every life story is unique but representative of every other life story, but clearly, more than one case should be considered, because as this review has indicated, there are various *types* of narrative to be considered.

What is being used as evidence here is, predominantly, research narratives, not therapeutic narratives or those constructed by interaction for a particular practical purpose, and not literary ones. An attempt is being made to combine the specificity of the total individual interview, its structure and context, with the generalisation that can perhaps be achieved by dissecting out various similarities or differences across a range of examples.

The purpose of the study (Blaxter and Poland 2002) from which these are taken was to elicit life and health histories in an exploration of issues related to the concept of social capital. This context must, of course, be noted. However, social capital was not introduced as a topic of conversation in these interviews, and they are as far as possible the freely volunteered accounts of lifelong health, with the interviewer intervening only to encourage the story along or sometimes clarify details. The 35 respondents were purposively selected on grounded theory principles, beginning with a group of elderly people living alone in a poor council estate, and broadening out for specific comparisons to others who were middle-aged rather than elderly, or not alone, or more prosperous, or living elsewhere in both urban and rural environments. Those who were elderly and in poor circumstances were of course likely to emphasise illness, but there were also younger people and those who perceived themselves as in excellent health, as well as some with chronic conditions. The interviews, tape-recorded, were of two hours or more and almost all conducted in the home; the respondents were simply told that we were interested in their ideas about their health, their life histories, and their environment.

They were encouraged to begin with their childhood and come up to the present time. Some few were not only articulate but well organised and with the narrator in control ('Alan', a sales consultant of 56, said firmly at one point: 'I think we'd better go through the rest of my history first and then it will fall into place') but more were circular and erratic and in places confused about the timing of events.

These are not *the* narratives of these individuals' lives, but *a* narrative – one of many they could tell, though it is perhaps assumed that all would bear some relationship to each other. Each of the narratives selected for discussion had a unique 'theme', a core statement about their identity running through the whole account. It would not be appropriate, though, to present them as *only* examples of one theme. Each demonstrated connections to other topics of the literature, and in each case issues of form, genre, structure and style are relevant.

The health and illness narratives

Jill: I've got a much more honest evaluation of what I am

Jill, a professional women of 45 living in the city, was articulate, conscious of her own identity, and presented herself as essentially responsible for her own troubled health history. She traced her personality – anxious, perfectionist, over-conscientious – to 'real complications with my childhood, which have affected me since then'. Both parents suffered from illness and though 'at the time I appeared to cope very well', 'it probably has affected my health long-term'. Distinct 'stories' recounted the experience of depression in her youth. Repetitive Strain Injury ended a career and resulted in registration as disabled, and ultimately, twenty years ago, she developed ME.

Her 'stories' of these illnesses were all tales of ups and downs, always accepted as her own responsibility which became part of her identity. Asked about the beginning of ME, she said, 'Stress. It started with a viral infection that I tried to fight through while I was under stress – massive, massive overwork.' At one time, 'I was pretty strong at that stage . . .', and at another 'It was always overwork when I do too much'. Some 'stories' were of times when her health was 'absolutely great' because she was happy: 'I was very, very fit. I had been used to looking after myself and used to not feeling supported by people around me'. Then there was the 'story' of 'the beginning of the end' with a new and responsible job ten years before, and another of being forced to stop work completely three years ago: 'When I do things I tend to be quite good at them, and people say you're good at that, and I think I am kind of hooked on the praise, actually . . . I pushed myself over the limit'. Some environmental causes were tentatively suggested, but '90 per cent of it was total overwork', causing the immune system to 'pack up' and a resultant diagnosis of 'extreme immune malfunction'. Throughout the latter part of the interview alternative and revised etiologies for her condition are offered: bad gastric flu, entero-viruses, a particular episode of exposure to pesticides, as well as stress and overwork. Only towards the end it emerged that Jill's sister, who was presented as sharing not only her family history but her personality, also had ME.

Jill explicitly tried to take the narrative into the future: 'I don't want to go back to working like that. At the same time it would be nice to be able to do fulfilling work again, and I'm not sure that I'll be able to. We'll see.' At the same time the narrative is one of change and reconciliation at the end:

> The people I used to work with . . . in some ways I am healthier than them even though I am not able to work. My physical health has collapsed completely, but in some ways my priorities are better.

[What makes you healthier?]

> Understanding yourself. If you've got ME and you've had it for years, you have to do some pretty hard and honest thinking about yourself . . . I always used to value myself in terms of what I could do. Now that I can't do anything that is of any use to anybody I think I've got a much more honest evaluation of what I am.

Susan: I'm responsible for me

The account of Susan, a divorced women of 52, living in an owner-occupied house in the country, was an interesting comparison because it was one of positive health, not illness. Her only 'problem' as a child – dyslexia – affected her academic achievement, but 'I just adopted that into me, my personality', and her subsequent life, through varied jobs, a failed marriage, and eventually a mature entry into a profession, was presented as entirely her own responsibility, her own independent choice. This was a clear example of (self-conscious) interaction between identity and (good) health. At various times she said 'I've never had any illness'; 'You have to keep a sense of identity'; and 'I've always got a sense that I'm responsible for me'. Of her failed marriage, she said:

> I thought I'd take my children and go.

[And how do you think it affected your health?]

> I think it made my health – just this sense of freedom, a sense that you're not oppressed. Your life isn't structured in this way and repressed ... The lifestyle was awful, the women [who were neighbours] just seemed to be miserable and depressed ... It was a surge of energy, you were on your own, you were making your own life.

In a sub-narrative of the type Jordens (2001) called 'observation', she talked at length about rural life, and the way in which it is conducive to health, because 'it allows you to be relaxed in your own body'. Asked, in conclusion, what she thought good health was, she gave an eloquent reply which was in the form of a generalisation, but in the light of her life story was obviously referring to herself:

> I think it's when some aspect of your needs is blocked, a channel is almost blocked, and all the needs you've got for your food and drink and your sexual needs and your emotional and artistic needs. They're in everyone, and they don't have to be filled to their absolute maximum, but it's very difficult to live with an imbalance ... If you're never allowed, if all you're given is your food and drink and no creativity comes into your life, no colour, you're never allowed to choose what you wear, it leads eventually to a dulling and you stop trying ... In general we haven't got a healthy attitude to all sorts of aspects of our lives, very blocked off.

Gerry – we all suffer from stress

Gerry, 54, was a local authority clerical worker, whose narrative flow shows strong counter currents flowing back and forwards through his account, currents of victim/but coping, healthy/but afraid of ill health, self-responsible/but under attack by irresistible forces, all bound up with moral and social (and especially masculine) identity. Initially, he claimed excellent health: 'I've probably been at the doctors five times in the last ten years', with any ailments explained away by accidental or environmental causes, such as bronchitis because of air pollution as a child. Gerry was one of the few respondents in this study who chose to situate talk about health in social and political contexts, however, and long digressions – at first, impersonal – were introduced. These were not 'stories' about himself, but more allied perhaps to what Bury called 'core' narratives, invoking deeper cultural levels of meaning. They were all about 'stress':

> We all suffer from stress, it's probably the biggest killer of all. Some of us cope with stress and some of us don't

and the failure of the moral fabric of our society . . .

> . . . people who are less strong than I am, they might just do away with themselves. The sheer despair of it.

General talk of stress seemed to be a deliberate introduction to, eventually, the events of his life which he presented as most harming his health, introduced suddenly with:

> . . . losing my one-year old, that was the biggest problem, her moving out with her mother, that was the hardest, the most stress of all.

Subsequently long separate 'stories' began to be inserted – of his divorce, his business failures, bankruptcy, claimed victimisation at work – interspersed with descriptions of 'society today': 'You have to try and fight, the strongest survive'. The themes are notably about coping as a *man* in a society where gender roles are changing:

> Health is a state of mind, about knowing what to do and how to do it, how to cope.

Another phase of the narrative talked of his own health in the present, with the first chinks in the optimistic presentation he had begun with:

It's harder when you get to this age, you haven't got the determination and willpower; You probably die sooner than you should if you're not exercising ...

(but on the other hand you should not push yourself, for)

... if you're a lazy fat whatsit like me you'll probably live longer because you're not pushing every bone in your body; I'm lucky because I've got to 54. A lot of men are known to have strokes, between the ages of 39 and 51 being the danger zone. I know my facts and figures.

He speculated more explicitly about his future than most respondents, and precisely in terms of what his identity will be: 'The future is bad because I can't see myself'. On the other hand, he listed health-promoting actions he meant to take, but always returning to the stress of his personal situation and how difficult change will be: 'Loneliness is the biggest killer of this century, believe me'. But then, in another turn, he disassociated himself from this helpless attitude:

The more you are out and occupied the less you think about the bad things that happen, it's the way to cope. You have to have hopes, dreams, and ambition. I still want to achieve.

Bill: I am a survivor

Bill, an active, independent and friendly man of 82 living in sheltered accommodation, had been a telephone linesman and engineer. Within the first five minutes of the interview he had mentioned that he spent three-and-a-half years in a Japanese prisoner-of-war camp:

That's why I think I've lasted more than most people because I'm alive after that sort of life ... I had dengue fever, a touch of malaria, diphtheria, and I survived the lot ... When we came home we went before a psychiatrist, just to see if we were mad I suppose [gleeful chuckle] – at least I'm certified sane!

This is an example of a whole health narrative organised around one turning point, an identity formed by an experience. This was a surprisingly common pattern, but notable in Bill's case because so long ago and apparently so forcefully expressed through the whole of his life. There was no vivid 'story', no description of the POW years (perhaps for the same reason he gave for not going on POW reunions – 'it's too upsetting') but the theme was pervasive throughout the interview. He returned time and again to this wartime experience. For instance, asked about 'healthy behaviour', he said:

Well, in the prison camp we used to smoke ... and ... the time I drank most was in the Army.

Asked what he thought about diet, he said:

I must say that's the one thing that has been left as a memory. I love food!

Like others, this respondent had a few words repeated throughout: discipline, responsibility, activity, (un)selfishness, independence. He said:

When we came home they told us to get on with our lives and that was it ... we were brought up for discipline.

And he used an interpretation of a hard, simple, and disciplined childhood, when communities were close and caring, to explain what a healthy life was like ('That's a different world today, everyone is self'). Bill represented his health as 'good, I can't complain', and had to be pressed for an account of actual health events, which in view of his years and hard working life might be expected to be numerous. Always they were minimised:

I got my leg gashed up, but you don't count that; I broke my neck twice, but that's just odds and ends; I'm deaf, of course (but 'I didn't do anything about it for some time – it's too much bother – I'm afraid I don't bother about things myself'); I had this fall [in his 80s] and I couldn't move my arm for nearly six months. I thought I'd try and cure this myself. But I had to go to the doctor in the end.

Vera: it's all about confidence and nerves

Vera, 75, a widow who had lived in the same council flat for 40 years, told a story of difficulty and failure, without clear resolution. Her 'nervous' identity and 'poor' health were intertwined since childhood.

I've had a lot of trouble with my nerves. I was so shy. I'm still the same. I never had any confidence, I still haven't got any, no confidence whatsoever.

The events of her life were told in a series of vivid short stories, not in any particular order but randomly as one thing prompted another. The first story was in childhood when she had diphtheria at nine, and remembered not being able to cry for her parents when in hospital:

You might be in trouble, I was always frightened of causing trouble.

At school, she 'was always too frightened to learn anything' and said that she deliberately 'failed' the 11+ 'because that would mean I was among strangers again'. Her youth during the war was described as lonely, because all her friends went into the forces:

> I always wanted to but I was too frightened to.

She lost a youthful boyfriend during the war:

> ... because he was going in for officer training, and you needed some- one different, his mother said I wasn't good enough.

One of the few stories concerning her subsequent marriage concerned believ- ing she was pregnant and her terror because 'I knew I couldn't manage on the money he gave me'.

The episodes of actual ill health that intervened were usually, however, attributed to external causes. She did join a woman's Service, but left after three days because she 'collapsed with the heat' on a parade ground. She worked in a factory where 'I was always having tonsillitis from the fumes from the batteries', and in shoe manufacturing where there was also pollut- ing material: 'that could be why I am breathless now'. There was a new job in her 50s which she found difficult to manage. The story of how 'at my time of life I couldn't see how I could change' went on for many pages of tran- script, leading up to a hospitalised 'breakdown'.

Her health at the present time was perceived as very poor, with glaucoma, chest complaints, sleeplessness and panic attacks. Asked to comment gen- erally on the things that had affected her health, her constantly repeated theme was the difficulties of her own character:

> It's all this, about confidence and nerves, it's been there all my life ... I think it was the feeling I'd always had about I couldn't do anything ... My sister and brother had families, and I'd never had any children. They were able to drive cars and I couldn't. There was always the feeling that I couldn't do anything.

Vera was articulate and interesting, eager to tell her narrative, but finally she said:

> You'd never believe the way I'm gassing on this afternoon, but I have a lot of trouble knowing what to talk to people about. I'm always afraid of that, you know, when you're waiting for them to say something, and you can't think of anything to talk about. That's hard really, but my life is so empty there's nothing to talk about.

Sarah: that was when I took charge of my life

Sarah, 74, lived alone in a council flat in a poor area. She described an early life of contentment in a poor childhood as one of seven children. She had not wanted to 'try for Grammar School' (although a brother had achieved this) because 'my parents couldn't afford the uniform', but an aunt had said 'let her have the chance' and offered to pay. However, at 17

> ... my mother did put the brakes on me when I started thinking about staying on and going to University – 'we've kept you there this long and we're just telling you it's time you were out in the world and earning'.

She described her subsequent life, working in offices, as 'I just drifted through life', healthy and content but without ambition and without putting effort into anything:

> It isn't anything to *do* to be healthy like that, it is? It's something that's in you, we're all individuals, I know, but it's just something that's in you

Again, she 'just drifted' into marriage, finding herself with a violent and selfish husband, and, eventually, several children:

> But I couldn't keep up any sort of hatred, you just got to get on with your living.

The rhythm of this story was regular and quiet. There was a constant theme of passivity, drifting, doing what was expected of her, with little self-aware-ness or feeling of self-worth. The narrative came to life and dealt with health only with dramatic 'stories' of the births of her children.

The narrative suddenly took a different rhythm and tone in her thirties, after the birth of her last child. Now she began to talk of feelings, to associ-ate them with health, and to tell stories in emotive language and at length:

> Then it clicked in my brain there's only one person who's going to look after you, your husband won't, so you'll have to look after yourself.

Her identity still centred around her role and duty as mother:

> It makes me look like an idiot for staying with him, but I suppose I had a very definite sort of feelings that my children had to know their father, know him and all his faults, that was the only way they were going to avoid making the same mistakes themselves.

She thought her husband would not tolerate the idea of her sterilisation, but her doctor offered her the contraceptive pill: 'And so I thought I better go on the pill as long as he doesn't know'. She summarized her life, at this age of 33:

> ... and that was what changed my life completely, because that was when I took charge of my life, wasn't it.

She did not finally leave her husband until age 58, talking of health in the meantime only in relation to her female roles (stress, side effects of the pill). Eventually, however:

> ... and really, I mean that was when my life sort of opened up ... once the children were grown up, I felt free to go.

Now, she presented herself as a self-reliant and independent individual, and healthy.

Terry: Going down the no-hopers route

At the end of this interview, Terry, a technician of 59 living with his second wife, when asked 'what the best part of his life' was, talked romantically and nostalgically of his early childhood in vivid detail ('I can't remember it ever raining') and also of his service in the Army and the early years of his first marriage. This was despite the fact that he had talked for some two hours about how his life had been one of tragedy and being defeated in his plans at every turn. Meningitis interfered with his schooling and meant his 'going down the no-hopers route'; he was diagnosed as epileptic and had to leave the Army; his divorce and the disputed paternity of his children were bitter episodes; there was continuous conflict with his mother who 'always tried to run my life'. He described his life in youth and during his first marriage as a fight against the label of epilepsy (though he experienced, apparently, only two seizures and had no stories of definite stigma to tell):

> I just felt that it was something sitting over the top of me, holding me back from doing what I wanted to.

Throughout, there were clear repeated expressions of loss, fear of illness, and inability to cope:

> I couldn't see any way forward at that time ... I couldn't see any future in anything ... I was withdrawing more and more into my shell.

His stories were all of episodes of medical terror: the first epileptic collapse, being threatened with a lumbar puncture when he had 'a very odd form of glandular fever', being hospitalised on another occasion, when he

> called the doctor, I think I've got meningitis

and

> I remember thinking she [doctor] didn't know what she was talking about, I'm dead, I'm definitely dying, I know it.

His story of his ill health *was* his life and his identity:

> How I handle everything, if that's really bad, I don't think about it.

Several times he returned to his early life, but retelling the story of meningitis rather than that of epilepsy. He presented himself now, however, at the time of interview, as come (in part with the aid of a Church) into calmer waters, and now relatively 'healthy'.

Sandra: love and affection bring you health

Sandra, 46, and a part-time school assistant living with her children and husband, offered an account of health wholly organised around the concept of motherhood. Her own mother 'couldn't cope', and Sandra looked after several siblings from an early age, taking two sisters (who called her Mum) to live with her when she married. She had four children of her own, and all talk of health turned to her family:

> I try to give my children different to what I had ... You've got to teach your kids the way to bring up, I know our mother didn't but we've got to teach our kids.

She was also still involved with her own parents, for though

> the doctor said, stay away from your mother, it's your mother that's making your health the way it is ... someone had to do it, it's on my shoulders again, she's still your mother!

Her own summary of her life was

> For 40 years all I've done is look after kids.

This narrative was not the linear one presented here, but circling, reiterating, moving backwards and forwards from her own family to her family of origin. But the theme was very clear: her health and her identity were defined in terms of mother-child relationships, and this was all she chose to discuss. There was no mention of her environment, except as part of her childhood, or of work, or of health-related behaviours – and incidentally, no mention of her husband. Her embedded stories were all about child-rearing, or her own daughters' pregnancies, and health events emerged only by-the-way: a damp bedroom as a child leading to lifelong rheumatism, high blood pressure after childbirth, or 'thyroid trouble' mentioned only half-way through a second hour of tape. Always she emphasised the importance of childhood and parental relationships:

> Love and affection bring you health, especially if you're happy in your childhood you're a fit person.

Her concept of health was not to do with disease, but a functional one related to these duties of daughter and mother:

> Health is being healthy in yourself, being fit, you've got to be fit in yourself to do things.

Themes and identities: narratives and stories

These narratives, like others in the research literature, each tend to have a particular theme, and these themes are clearly connected to identity. Bill's theme was one of survivorship, Terry's of defeat, Susan's of self-responsibility, and Vera's of lack of self-confidence. The whole narrative is saying 'this is who I am'. It seems likely that these are habitual stories – 'this is how I always think of myself' – but occasionally there was the sense of some construction of this presentation actually occurring during the interview. Ideas of cause presented tentatively and diffidently at one point, with much use of the word 'perhaps', become repeated later as definite 'facts'.

There is no assumption that people are so crudely identified, whether to themselves or an audience, in one-word themes. Simply, the narrative form appears to require a themed presentation. In part, it is the strain towards making a coherent whole of life. But health is the category of events that people are being asked to talk about, and it is not surprising that health becomes entirely bound up with their 'normal' presentation of the self.

It is notable that it is the stories-within-narratives that most clearly express the individual theme. It is possible for life and health to be described in what Bury called contingent narratives, the telling of discrete events just as they happened, whether or not they are remembered in sequence or jumbled into random choices of what might be relevant – what Kirmayer

(2000) calls 'broken narratives', fragile, incomplete and inconsistent. In the narratives used here, however, wherever 'stories' intervene, the themes immediately become clear. Thus Jill's stories, whether of particular happy times of her life when her health had been good, or episodes of different sorts of ill health, were all about the relationship of her personality to her health. Terry's stories were vivid accounts of different illness episodes from childhood onwards, all with a theme of defeat and helplessness. Vera similarly told a series of different stories – childhood illness 65 years before, wartime youth, several different types of work experience – which all had the theme of fear and inadequacy. Sandra's stories, though not explicitly involving much introspection about her own character, were without exception on the topic of the roles of daughter and of mother. Another respondent, Don (whose narrative is not given), in every story of an illness, returned to childhood and his relationship with his father. Riessman (1990) similarly showed in the narrative of a man with advanced multiple sclerosis how the speaker breaks the frame set by the research interview to create themed 'narrative enclaves' within the discourse – stories, in this case, in each of the roles of husband, father and worker, which served to define his identity.

This type of narrative, where there seemed to be two separate activities going on, the life narrative and the embedded illustrative story, was not universal in the examples given here. Gerry and Susan were two respondents whose longest 'virtuoso' passages were less openly personal, presented more as the offering of strongly-held opinions. In general, however, it appeared that this use of stories was the feature of the narrative form which made the relationship of health and identity most clear.

Structures of identity: past, present and future

The essential feature of a narrative is that it has to have a plot: a past, present and future. This temporal sequence is what gives it meaning – events which are scattered in time, a seemingly random sequence, become a logical whole. Most often, this relates to 'who I have been and am and may become', that is, to identity. The life narrative relates to the 'internal subjective sense of having a life story that organises our understanding of our past life, our current situation, and our imagined future' (Linde 1993: 11).

It is a commonplace observation that health narratives reorganise and reconstruct the past, straining always to connect, to present a health history as a chain of cause and effect. In the light of the present, the past is rewritten in an attempt to achieve what Pinder (1992) called 'experiential coherence'. As Mattingly (1994) suggested, we make as well as tell stories, and narratives are not altogether lived before they are told.

Research which can actually demonstrate this rewriting of the past is not common, though one study (Blaxter and Paterson 1982) did have the opportunity to compare health stories (of childbearing and child care) with contemporary accounts of 25 years before, to find that they were (almost certainly involuntarily) often an erratic match. More frequently, the process can be demonstrated by inconsistencies and re-tellings in a long interview. The present sheds light on the past: 'I must have been like this, in order to be as I am now', 'The beginning of this was then, though I did not recognise it at the time'.

This rewriting links events temporarily, when in reality they were more discrete. The women studied by Blaxter and Paterson (1982) clearly rewrote and re-ordered their histories, and not only their own but also their families' through several generations. The idea of illness happening quite randomly and with different causes at different times seemed to be uncomfortable: they much preferred to see their health and their lives as continuous logical wholes, where this illness 'went into' that, and this disease had its roots in events years or even generations before. The way in which this was interpreted was a liking for continuity, a desire to assert their identities. In circumstances of deprivation, with little material success to boast of, their histories of close families represented their wealth and identity. Other studies have similarly noted the reordering of the past as an explanation of the present. Riessman (1990), for instance, described how a respondent linked a diagnosis of MS to his divorce, though the events were separated by nine years. Frank (1997), using published illness narratives, gave examples of the way in which illness symptoms 'unlocked the past', raising memories which might or might not be 'really' related to the present but nevertheless provided attachments weaving the illness into identity. People may in fact realise what they are doing: as one respondent said: 'The brain wants to make order of what happened to me. It wants to have experience make sense, no matter what kind of mental gymnastics we have to go through' (Garro 1994: 779).

In the data used here, Jill – as is common in accounts of disputed diagnoses such as ME – clearly looked for alternative etiologies in the past, trying to produce a coherent story-line. Terry's and Sandra's accounts were both composed of a linked series of health events since youth, all situated within family relationships and events. Sally, one of the respondents whose narrative was not summarised here, gave a long and vivid account of an eventful and troubled life, explicitly reinterpreting the past at every stage:

> Looking back, I think [son] was a sickly child because I didn't have the right food when I was pregnant ... My health really went down [after an abusive marriage], I only see that now, it erodes away your self-confidence.

As the past is re-valued, so the future is hypothesised. A narrative must have an end, otherwise it cannot have a time trajectory. The future is often the dimension to which least space is given in the narrative, but it could be argued that the (usually) uncertain end-point is always there, pulling the narrative flow along, even if implicitly:

> If the meaning of the present, and even of the past, is contingent on what unfolds in the future, then what is happening and what has happened is not a matter of fact but of interpretive possibilities which are vulnerable to an unknown future (Mattingly 1994: 820).

The search for an end is commonly ambiguously expressed, because the possibility of different endings has to be maintained (DelVecchio Good *et al.* 1994). Perceptions of health at some future time, as a self which is changing, developing, coping, achieving or being destroyed, depend on health experience through the whole of life. Lawton (2002), asking people to think specifically about perceptions of self and health at some future date, found that seeing the self as vulnerable and the future as contingent depended on lifetime experience of severe or chronic illness.

The concept of emplotment in therapy suggests that horizons have to be blurred, and stages carefully calibrated, in order to allow patients to live in the immediate world. The future narrative is about struggle, hope and progress. But, in personal narratives rather than clinical ones, these coexist with other, unspoken narratives about the future: what Bruner (1986) called 'subjunctivising reality' or trafficking in possibilities. People play end-games or create an as-if. This is exemplified in the book-length narrative of cancer analysed by Crossley (2003), where the fear of death is exorcised by breaking down the future into ever smaller units. Where the future is difficult to see, what Herzlich (1973) called 'illness as occupation' is perhaps a way of dealing with it; as a respondent of Garro (1994: 783) said:

> All I do twenty-four hours a day is work on my health, think about what else, what am I overlooking, what could I do, what could I try.

Among the narratives being considered here, the past, present and future were clearly separated as dimensions of identity in Gerry's case, even though it progressed tangent by tangent rather than in a logical linear form. There was the tale of the past, when he was a victim, unable to cope, suffering the pressures of what he saw as societal trends over which he had no control; in the present he presented himself as more positively involved in that society and no longer in such conflict with it; he had doubts about the future but speculated on a new identity. Jill was another respondent who staged the past and present clearly, and explicitly took the narrative into the future, insisting that she had reached a new plateau of ability and a new evaluation of herself from which she could go forward. Terry's narrative was another that dealt almost exclusively on a 'regressive' story of the past, but at the end looked to the possibility of a degree of change in himself and a more hopeful future.

Biographical disruption

Since these are not narratives of *an* illness, but of the health events throughout life – good health and bad health, 'ordinary' illness and chronic disease – they may be interesting to consider in the context of 'biographical disruption'. Bury (1982: 170), in particular, has discussed how chronic illness can cause a disruption in peoples' lives 'such that a fundamental rethinking of the person's biography and self-concept is involved'. Narrative makes it possible to give meaning to disruptive events that change not only the course of life but also who one is. In Hydén's phrase, narrative offers the opportunity 'to knit together the split ends of time, to construct a new context and fit the illness disruption into a temporal framework' (1997: 53).

A great many studies have demonstrated this. Charmaz (1983) described the loss of self, but how the self then undergoes change in order to regain continuity of identity. Corbin and Strauss (1987) suggested that biography has three dimensions, biographical time, conception of body and conception of self, and when the conceptual chain between these is broken by the advent of a chronic illness, narrative has to be used to put it back together. Williams (1984), Bury (1988) and Kleinman (1988) all showed how the experience of chronic pain or severe illness caused a revision of life goals, but how patients nevertheless maintained a sense of self.

Several of the narratives discussed here might have involved biographical disruption. Jill's, in particular, was the description of the development and eventual diagnosis of ME, a typical topic in this genre. Several others related health events long before which were remembered as life-changing, such as Terry's meningitis and diagnosis of epilepsy.

There were also distinct biographical disruptions, what Frank (1995) called aporias, or tears in the fabric of lives, in the stories of Sarah, Susan or Gerry. The impression given by these narratives, however, is more of knitting or holding the fabric of life together, more of continuity in identity than change. The disruptions were more likely to be described as the *cause* of changes in health, not the result of health events. Though Jill's ME did disrupt her life, she was clear that it did not change her identity. Health and identity were connected long before the advent of the chronic disease, and her narrative is, rather, one of a very stable self which persisted through good health and bad. It cannot, of course, be judged how far this is the rewriting described by Bury, but this and other narratives would seem to suggest that the acute sense of biographical disruption impacting on identity in many chronic illness studies may be particular to research on coming to terms with disease.

Moral identities

Narratives are structured by the speaker for a purpose, and if they are not given an obvious one by the research situation they will usually create one. As Goffman (1961) had noted in *Encounters*, they are usually social apologia, either success stories or stories distancing a failed life from individual blame. The basic plot is a moral one, explaining, reconstructing, and negotiating the value of life. Accounts of health and illness, in particular, are as Radley and Billig (1996) suggested, claims to be worthy individuals, fit participants in the social world. Because the notion of ill health as deviance is pervasive, the presentation of health becomes a moral pursuit and illness narratives become 'moral ethnographies' (Charmaz 1991) showing how patients make moral decisions about their identity.

Those who are ill have a particular need to legitimate themselves. Examples of this in the literature include, for instance, the narrative of a rheumatoid arthritis sufferer of Williams (1993), stressing her autonomy, adaptation, personal control and good sense. Threats to autonomy drew her actively into the pursuit of virtue in the form of the avoidance of uncleanliness and dependence. Riessman (1990) similarly demonstrated how narratives of illness are essentially sustaining a positive definition of the self – 'enclaves' are inserted into the account to assert an identity which might contrast with some of the realities of the situation, an identity which is disabled but still a good worker, unable to interact with a son but still a good father.

The presentation of self as healthy can equally be a moral enterprise, showing good health to be the result of a strong or virtuous identity. Susan's narrative of health, though often elaborated in an impersonal and generalised way, was essentially a moral claim: attitudes, and in particular, the free flow of creative and artistic impulses, were the definition of the healthy identity. Sandra's was also a moral narrative of the achievement of health through the quest to be a good daughter and mother. It could be argued that the commonly noted tendency to claim good health even in the face of evidence to the contrary is essentially a moral claim. This was noted particularly in the women's narratives of Blaxter and Paterson (1982) of lives spent in socially deprived circumstances. These had almost inevitably poor health histories, but the women presented a very culturally distinct 'just deserts' view of illness. Hard work equalled virtue, and health was the reward of virtue, so that denying ill health or refusing to 'lie down' to it were claims to a virtuous life. In the narratives used here, Bill's was clearly an example of some conflict between subjective presentation and objective clinical facts. He did admit to some of the ills of old age, but his belittling of them and insistence on his excellent health were part of a moral presentation of identity as independent, disciplined and self-reliant. It would be inappropriate, of course, to use the word 'presentation' in any dismissive sense, for he had actually developed an identity which was continually worked out in the details of his daily behaviour.

For those for whom it is impossible to sustain an identity of essential healthiness, the narrative can still be used to justify moral identity. Terry's was clearly the justification of a life which had not gone as successfully as he might have hoped. Illness had interfered, through no fault of his own, with a self that might have been more in control, been better able to do 'what I wanted to'. Past illnesses – even long past, in childhood – were the grounds for his fearfulness throughout life. Don was another respondent whose whole history was devoted to justifying the lack of the straightforward career his parents had expected of him. A long series of stories of stressful incidents served to explain how poor health was both the cause and the result of the person he had become.

Serious illness may not be possible to deny, but at least it offers an opportunity for the ill person to rise to the occasion. As Frank (1997) discussed, however, there is a fundamental problem in that most of the situations ill people face may admit no single 'really right thing': the question may be 'who might I become to resolve this issue?' At the best, they may become the sort of person who can live with a less than satisfactory solution. Coping with ill health, being 'successfully' ill, may restore virtue. The self is the means for fighting illness, as Jill's narrative showed, and if one cannot fight, as Vera expressed clearly, the self is flawed.

A major feature of health and illness narratives is their extremely common emphasis on speculation of cause and effect, which is often a kind of moral testing. In the narratives of the women of Blaxter (1983) there was obvious trying-out of causes in one's own behaviour (admitting 'that's smoking, of course' or blaming self-neglect) and those which were external and inevitable ('in my circumstances, I could not have acted differently'). This is often a dialogue with the self, as much as with the listener: Hydén (1995), for instance, describes a psychiatric patient whose narrative explored the extent to which he himself was responsible – was his illness the result of too high expectations of self, or attempts to live up to the expectations of his mother, or was it wholly inherent in his identity because inherited? The patients of Garro (1994) were seen as being susceptible to a psychological model of etiology, but since attributing ill health to the mind rather than the body meant a suggestion of inadequacy and blame, this set up a dilemma for the presentation. Garro's respondents, it was suggested, dealt with this by defining cause in terms of 'my body's response to stress', thus separating mind and body, or identity and the events which impinged on it. This seems to be a common moral stratagem. In the present series, Gerry's narrative was a clear example of a dialogue back and forth between attitude and behaviour, fighting and coping, stress and the pressures of society, as influencing his past, present and future health.

Narratives of social identity

Discussion of health narratives and identity tends naturally to focus on the individual – the events of a particular life and their interaction with a personality. Every individual is a part of a reference group with its own history, however, and cannot be separated from it. The collective past is also relevant. Health events take place in a context of generational cohorts, occupational identity, social class and local history. These also are narratives in time, incorporating specific cultural meanings and affected by social change.

Herzlich and Pierret (1987), in particular, studied how the 'collective representation' of 'the modern way of life' shapes the understanding of an illness. Sontag (1977) had rejected a view of cancer as situated in identity, seeing this as a moralising blame placed on the individual, but the respondents of Herzlich and Pierret spoke of it as a psychic illness caused by modern life: an illness produced by society, but manifesting itself in the flaws of modern identity.

There are many other examples in the literature of the importance of social identity. Brock and Kleiber (1994) described how athletes incorporated sports injury narratives into their identity *as* an athlete: injury threatened this identity, but by stressing the cause of the injury they confirmed their attachment to a particular reference group. Carricaburu and Pierret (1995) showed how for haemophiliac and gay respondents HIV changed both work and relationships, but for both could at the same time reinforce an identity. For everyone, severe illness is likely to provide revised versions of social roles, but these new roles are bound to particular times and places. Hunt (2000), for instance, showed how Mexican patients being treated for a cancer that results in gender liminality actively constructed a new identity specific to their own culture.

Skultans (1999) has offered particularly well developed analyses of the way in which historical events are 'annexed to the body' and used to explain the development of mental illness. The narrative of a Latvian countrywoman was offered as a testament of the violence and injustice of past experience: 'Bodily experience plays a central role as a yardstick against which the unreasonableness of history is judged' (Skultans 1999: 310). In another analysis, Skultans (2003) emphasised the movement from the somatic to psychological language of distress in a particular culture, and how these changes link to 'ideas of agency, victimhood and shared versus private articulations of pain.' In contrast to an earlier era of the culture where disorder and lack of predictability were attributed to society, now the narratives showed internalised values of an enterprise culture and personal responsibility.

In the study of the liver disease patients (Blaxter and Cyster 1984) there were several narratives of this disease which (because of its association with alcohol and lifestyles) were as much accounts of a particular culture and period as of individuals. For instance, a man telling stories of his life as a fisherman in a disappearing industry and depressed area, characterised for generations by the hard drinking that was the mark of group membership and masculinity, was not denying his own responsibility for his health history. He was, however, describing how his society – and his identity – had changed over a historical period from one which was strong and in control to one which was without health or hope.

In the Blaxter and Poland (2002) sample the oldest generation were perhaps the last for whom the historical event of the Second World War was the defining event of their lives, affecting not only their identity but their lifelong health. It was something they talked of at length, associating current health with the events so long before. Bill's was the most obvious example, but several others returned to wartime experience when discussing the general course of their health. Many of the patients of the liver disease study also related their disease, at least in part, to aspects of war service 40 years before, ranging from the social pressures to smoke and drink to the possibility of 'over-injections' and tropical infections.

One conspicuous aspect of many narratives was their emphasis on gender roles. That health was closely connected with male or female identity was not surprising, but for many it was social changes in gender relationships which were most closely linked to the history of their cohort on the one hand and the development of their individual health-history and identity on the other. Sarah's narrative was clearly a 'progressive' history of an identity conceived largely in terms of the conventional female role of her times ('He believed that was what women were for, you know, to do the housework and everything') until first her dawning of independence at 33 and the final 'opening up' of life at 58. All the illnesses she spoke of were associated with the female role, and her self-perceived good health since middle age was almost a metaphor for a new self. She never explicitly presented herself as a representative of her generation and class, and had a clear sense of individual personality as the driving force of her life. Nevertheless she did represent women who suffered before the rise of feminism (and the pill) and benefited from it. Susan more explicitly and impersonally associated the lives of women of her generation with their health. She was very conscious of the effects of women's roles, especially in circumstances of deprivation and lack of education:

> Those women who are the healthiest seem to be those women who have mostly got their marriage but have got their own interests throughout their lives, who have retained their own sense of identity. It's very hard

for a women, a girl, maybe more so in my day, to keep a sense of identity without serving other people.

Similarly, several men were greatly concerned to display or maintain their masculinity. Terry's relationship with his mother and partners, and his identity as a wage-earner and provider, were the main topics of his stories. The central theme of Gerry's narratives was the problem of 'coping as a man' in a changing society:

> More and more women are equal, there's nothing wrong with women being equal and achieving, but men aren't as necessary. Women can do all the jobs in the house now, what do they need a man for. We used to be superior – the whole thing has changed in the last 30 years ... men are going downhill because they are unnecessary ... We're a bankrupt nation, nobody cares, life has changed.

Don was another respondent who dwelt on the differences during his life-time in the balance of gender roles, but in his case it was welcomed because he had felt that the pressures on him as a provider had been responsible for his ill health.

Conclusion

This chapter has used some case histories, in the context of other literature, to consider the value of the life narrative as a means for exploring the relationship of health and identity. It has shown that people *do* construct life-long identities around their health and illness experiences, and their narratives centre around these images of themselves. In part, the process becomes visible through attention to form and structure, flow, pace and vocabulary, and in particular to the embedded 'stories'. Each episode – each health event and life period – can be categorised in ways described at the beginning of the chapter, as progressive, stable or regressive, as res-titution, quest or chaos, as ways of dealing with biographical disruption and above all occasions for the display of moral character.

Much of the sociological literature of chronic illness concerns the *effects* of health on the sufferer's identity: how people become struggling, or changed, or defeated, or surviving individuals. In another tradition, there is a literature of how personality or identity may be the *cause* of illness, or at least the determinant of the way in which it is interpreted or responded to. The notable impression of the narratives discussed here, however, was that – over a lifetime of good and bad health – health and identity were inextricably mixed.

The purpose for which a narrative is told must always be taken into account. There are obvious differences between interviews focusing on a particular disease or health event, and whole accounts of life. In narratives involving severe and chronic illness, a degree of reconstruction of self was evident. To some extent, the accounts had the obvious purposes of addressing personal and social conflicts, demonstrating competence, and legitimating a self whom the illness had not destroyed.

Where the narrative was a wider one, however, considering varied health and illness experiences throughout life, these experiences were presented largely as forming the identities which were being offered. There was a likelihood of these being childhood or early life events. Almost every narrative then placed a degree of responsibility for subsequent good or bad health on this personality and the lifestyle in which it was expressed. Respondents were saying: these events which were beyond my control made me the person I am; my relationship to my body and the world it inhabits explains my health. Thus the effects of health upon identity, and the effects of identity on health, could be seen as moving back and forth reciprocally throughout the narratives.

Finally, another point demonstrated in this review is that it seems important not to focus exclusively on individual identity. The narratives relate also to social groups, cohorts, eras and places. The interaction of gender roles, social history, and health was particularly obvious. As Kleinman (1988:31) noted, the health and illness which is summarised in these narratives soaks up not only personal but also social significance.

Acknowledgement

The study from which the narratives used here are taken was funded by the Health Development Agency. Fiona Poland, School of Occupational and Physical Therapy, University of East Anglia, was joint Principal Investigator, and acknowledgement must be made to Monica Curran who conducted the interviews.

References

Backett K. (1992) 'Taboos and excesses: lay health moralities in middle class families', *Sociology of Health and Illness*, 14, 2, 255–74.
Blaxter M. (1983) 'The causes of disease: women talking', *Social Science and Medicine* 1, 2, 59–69.
Blaxter M. (1993) 'Why do the victims blame themselves?' in A. Radley (ed.) *Worlds of Illness: Biographical and Cultural Perspectives on Health and Disease*, London, Routledge, 124–42.
Blaxter M. and Paterson E. (1982) Mothers and Daughters: A Three-generational Study of Health Attitudes and Behaviour, London, Heinemann.

Blaxter M. and Cyster R. (1984) 'Compliance and risk-taking: the case of alcoholic liver disease', *Sociology of Health & Illness*, 6, 3, 290–310.

Blaxter M. and Poland F. (2002) 'Moving beyond the survey in exploring social capital' in C. Swann and A. Morgan (eds) *Social capital for health, insights from qualitative research*, Health Development Agency.

Brock S.C. and Kleiber D.A. (1994) 'Narratives in medicine: the stories of elite college athletes' career-ending injuries', *Qualitative Health Research*, 4, 411–30.

Brody H. (1994) ' "My story is broken; Can you help me fix it?" Medical ethics and the joint construction of narrative', *Literature and Medicine*, 13, 1, 79–92.

Bruner J. (1986) *Actual Minds, Possible Worlds*, Cambridge, MA, Harvard University Press.

Bury M. (1982) 'Chronic illness as biographical disruption', *Sociology of Health and Illness*, 4, 2, 167–82.

Bury M. (1988) 'Meanings at risk: the experience of arthritis'in R. Anderson and M. Bury (eds) *Living with Chronic Illness: the Experience of Patients and their Families*, London, Unwin Hyman.

Bury M. (1991) 'The sociology of chronic illness: a review of research and prospects', *Sociology of Health and Illness*, 13, 451–68.

Bury M. (2001) 'Illness narratives: fact or fiction?', *Sociology of Health and Illness*, 23, 3, 263–85.

Carricaburu D. and Pierret J. (1995) 'From biographical disruption to biographical reinforcement: the case of HIV-positive men', *Sociology of Health and Illness*, 17, 1, 65–88.

Charmaz K. (1983) 'Loss of self: a fundamental form of suffering in the chronically ill', *Sociology of Health and Illness*, 5, 168–95.

Charmaz K. (1991) *Good days, bad days: the self in chronic illness and time*, New Brunswick, Rutgers University Press.

Corbin J. and Strauss A. (1987) 'Accompaniment of chronic illness changes in body, self, biography and biographical time', *Research in the Sociology of Health Care*, 6, 249–81.

Cornwell J. (1984) *Hard-earned lives: accounts of Health and Illness from East London*, London, Tavistock.

Crossley M.L. (2003) 'Let me explain': narrative emplotment and one patient's experience of oral cancer', *Social Science and Medicine*, 56, 3, 439–48.

Davison C., Frankel S. and Davey Smith G. (1992) 'The limits of lifestyle: re-assessing "fatalism" in the popular culture of illness prevention', *Social Science and Medicine*, 34, 6, 675–85.

DelVecchio Good M.-J., Munakata T., Kobayashi Y., Mattingly C. and Good B.J. (1994) 'Oncology and Narrative Time', *Social Science and Medicine*, 38, 6, 855–62.

Denzin N.K. (1986) 'Interpretive interactionism and the use of life histories', *Review of International Sociology*, 44, 321–37.

Elliott A. (2001) *Concepts of Self*, Cambridge, Cambridge Polity Press.

Frank A.W. (1995) *The Wounded Storyteller: Body, Illness and Ethics*, London, University of Chicago Press.

Frank A.W. (1997) 'Illness as moral occasion: restoring agency to ill people', *Health*, 1(2), 131–48.

Garro L.C. (1994) 'Narrative representations of chronic illness experience: cultural models of illness, mind, and body in stories concerning the temporomandibular joint (TMJ)', *Social Science and Medicine*, 38, 6, 775–88.

Goffman E. (1961) *Encounters*, Indianapolis, Bobbs-Merrell.

Good B.J. and DelVecchio Good M.-J. (1994) 'In the subjunctive mode: epilepsy narratives in Turkey', *Social Science & Medicine*, 38, 6, 835–42.

Hawkins A.H. (1990) ' change of heart: the paradigm of regeneration in medical and religious narrative', *Perspectives in Biology and Medicine*, 33, 547–59.

Herzlich C. (1973) *Health and Illness*, London, Academic Press.

Herzlich C. and Pierret J. (1987) *Illness Self and Society*, Baltimore, John Hopkins University Press.

Hunt L.M. (2000) 'Strategic suffering: Illness narratives as social empowerment among Mexican Cancer patients' in L.C. Garro and C. Mattingly (eds), *Narrative and the Cultural Construction of Illness and Healing*, University of California Press, 88–107.

Hydén L.-C. (1995) 'In search of an ending. Narrative reconstruction as a moral quest', *Journal of Narrative and Life History*, 5, 67–84.

Hydén L.-C. (1997) 'Illness and narrative', *Sociology of Health and Illness*, 19, 1, 48–69.

Jordens C.F.C., Little M., Paul K. and Sayers E.-J. (2001) 'Life disruption and generic complexity: a social linguistic analysis of narratives of cancer illness', *Social Science and Medicine*, 53, 9, 1227–36.

Kelleher D. (1988) *Diabetes*, London, Routledge.

Kelly M. and Dickenson H. (1997) 'The narrative self in autobiographical accounts of illness', *Sociological Review*, 45.2 254–78.

King N.M.P. and Stanford A.F. (1992) 'Patient stories, doctor stories, and true stories: a cautionary reading', *Literature and Medicine*, 11, 2, 185–99.

Kirmayer L.J. (2000) 'Broken narratives: Clinical encounters and the poetics of illness experience' in L.C. Garro and C. Mattingly (eds), *Narrative and the Cultural Construction of Illness and Healing*, Berkeley University of California Press, 153–80.

Kleinman A. (1988) *The Illness Narrative, Suffering, Healing and the Human Condition*, New York, Basic Books.

Lawton J. (2002) 'Colonising the future: temporal perceptions and health-relevant behaviours across the adult lifecourse', *Sociology of Health and Illness*, 24, 6, 714–33.

Linde C. (1993) *Life Stories and the Creation of Coherence*, Oxford, Oxford University Press.

Mathieson C.M. and Stam H.J. (1995) 'Renegotiating identity: cancer narratives', *Sociology of Health and Illness*, 17, 3, 283–306.

Mattingly C. (1994) 'The concept of therapeutic "emplotment"', *Social Science and Medicine*, 38, 6, 811–22.

McAdams D.P. (1989) 'The development of narrative identity' in D. M. Buss and N. Cantor (eds) *Personal Psychology: Recent Trends and Emerging Directions*, New York, Springer-Verlag, 160–74.

Pierret J. (1993) 'Constructing discourses about health and their social determinants' in A. Radley (ed.) *Worlds of Illness: Biographical and Cultural Perspectives on Health and Disease*, London, Routledge, 9–26.

Pinder R. (1992) 'Coherence and incoherence: doctors' and patients' perspectives on the diagnosis of Parkinson's Disease', *Sociology of Health & Illness*, 14, 1, 1–22.

Pollock K. (1993) 'Attitude of mind as a means of resisting illness' in A. Radley (ed.) *Worlds of Illness: Biographical and Cultural Perspectives on Health and Disease*, London, Routledge, 49–70.

Radley A. (1993) 'The role of metaphor in adjustment to chronic illness' in A. Radley (ed.) *Worlds of Illness: Biographical and Cultural Perspectives on Health and Disease*, London, Routledge, 109–23.

Radley A. and Billig M. (1996) 'Accounts of health and illness: dilemnas and representations', *Sociology of Health and Illness*, 18, 2, 220–40.

Riessman C.K. (1990) 'Strategic uses of narrative in the presentation of self and illness: a research note', *Social Science and Medicine*, 30, 11, 1195–200.

Robinson I. (1990) 'Personal narratives, social careers and medical courses: analysing life trajectories in autobiographies of people with multiple sclerosis', *Social Science and Medicine*, 30, 11, 1173–86.

Skultans V. (1999) 'Narratives of the body and history: illness in judgement on the Soviet past', *Sociology of Health & Illness*, 21, 3, 310–28.

Skultans V. (2003) 'From damaged nerves to masked depression: inevitability and hope in Latvian psychiatric narratives', *Social Science and Medicine* (in press).

Sontag S. (1977) *Illness as Metaphor*, New York, Farrar, Straus and Giroux.

Wikan U. (2000) 'With life in one's lap: The story of an eye/I (or two)' in L.C. Garro and C. Mattingly (eds), *Narrative and the Cultural Construction of Illness and Healing*, University of California Press, 212–36.

Williams G. (1984) 'The genesis of chronic illness: narrative reconstruction', *Sociology of Health and Illness*, 6, 175–200.

Williams G. (1993) 'Chronic illness and the pursuit of virtue in everyday life' in A. Radley (ed.) *Worlds of Illness: Biographical and Cultural Perspectives on Health and Disease*, London, Routledge, 92–108.

Conclusion

David Kelleher and Gerard Leavey

It may be true, as Bauman (2001) suggests, that identity has become a popular topic for sociologists, psychologists and literary critics to write about, but few have made the links between it and the range of illness conditions explored in this book. The links are also made between the nature of contemporary society, variously described as globalised, post-traditional, late modern and post-modern, disorganised capitalism and the importance taken on by individualism and identity. The experience of illness is described, in chapters on Alzheimer's, cancer, the pain experienced by professional rugby players and the opening chapter by Kelly and Millward on chronic illness and identity. Not all of the chapters explore links of this kind however. There are also chapters examining the links between religion and illness, religion as an alternative to psychiatry in the case of West African Pentecostalism (Leavey) and one linking the experience of emigration to the development of ill-health.

What is it about contemporary society, which makes it not only possible but also sensible to link these personal experiences to the nature of society? We need to expand on the descriptive terms used above to make the links. Those who write about society, variously described above, all include individualism as one of the key features of present day Western society, the decline of class solidarity and its replacement, to some extent, by the ephemeral life-style cultures lacking the cohesive groupings of yesterday. Individuals have to realise their own worlds, contribute to the making of their own present and future but to do this they have to reflexively understand their past. Otherwise, as Giddens (1991) notes;

> Personal meaningless – the feeling that life has nothing worthwhile to offer – becomes a fundamental psychic problem in circumstances of late modernity.
>
> (Giddens 1991: 9)

This may be particularly so for people facing the prospect of the removal of a breast or for people, through the experience of Alzheimer's, who fear losing control of their minds, facing chaos and holding onto the core of their identity and place in the world. The situation of women with breast cancer looking at how they might appear in the future without one of the characteristics defining their gender identity, is narrated with a sharp touch of humour in one of the interviews when a South Asian woman rebukes a male doctor who suggests that no one will notice the difference:

> I don't know what else he was saying. He must have been saying other things that I wasn't hearing. And that was it. It was like someone poked me with a needle and I jumped up two feet. I said, 'If someone took your thinga majig out and filled your underpants with plastic ... ?'

In a quite different way, the chapter on Sport, Health and Identity shows how professional rugby players nurse their slower and battered bodies through what is identified as a pre-retirement phase of their relatively short career in the limelight as they look towards the future. Sport for many people is not something they do professionally, of course, but as Scambler et al. point out, an activity they take up in pursuit of fitness and health, and, as in the case of the body builders in particular, in the pursuit of looking good and finding an identity in and beyond the gym. Bauman (op. cit.) makes the related point that 'we do not die or live as we are born' by quoting Jean-Paul Sartre who remarked that 'it is not enough to be born a bourgeois – one must live one's life as a bourgeois'. This makes the point, as do all the chapters in the book, that, 'How should I live?' is a question that people in this world without meta-narratives have constantly to ask themselves in their reflexive search for an authentic identity they can live with. As Mildred Blaxter says in her chapter in this book:

> Through narrative people rearrange their experience, present their actions for judgement, and come to articulate their situation in the world. Indeed, identity is a life story.

The situation of emigrants relates to one of the most often used descriptions of the contemporary world as being a globalised world with the consequent disembedding of populations and cultures. For people who have come from Bangladesh and even from rural Ireland the question of 'How should I live?' is a particularly pressing one every day. But it is also a question faced by others whose life is changed by chronic illness as the narratives in this book suggest. The world they, and we, live in is a world where cultural certainties are under challenge from the power of disorganised capital, which is able to override the power of national economies yet encourage ethnic differences while the differentiating traditions of how to live are in decline. Bauman (2001: 34) describes the globalised world as:

> ... processes seen as self-propelling, spontaneous and erratic, with no one sitting at the control desk and no one taking on planning, let alone taking charge of overall results.

No wonder that those struggling to face a future with a chronic illness have problems in fixing an identity.

References

Bauman Z. (2001) *The Individualised Society,* Cambridge, Polity Press.
Giddens A. (1991) *Modernity and Self-Identity,* Cambridge, Polity Press.

Index

ageism 62–3
Alzheimer, Alois 65
Alzheimer's disease 14, 59–60, 64–75
 advance directives 67
 anxieties 65–6
 awareness of self 66
 cultural perspectives 72–4
 effects on carers 69–70
 family considerations 68–70
 identity maintenance work 70
 research approaches 72
 social constructionist considerations
  67–8
 staff considerations 70–2
 symptoms 65
 wandering 72
Alzheimer's Society 64
Antenna 48–52
anti-Catholicism 84–5
anti-dementia drugs 74
aporias 190
asthma 138
authenticity 93
autoprosopagnosia 66

Ballymacross 129–30
 collective identity 132, 143, 144
 communal spirit 141, 143
 Protestants in 140
 see also Northern Ireland health study
belief systems 123–4
biographical disruption 8, 12–13, 190–1
bodily integrity, threatened by cancer
  26–31
body
 and identity 9–10
 maintenance of 109
 materiality of 28, 30

bodybuilding 110–12
breast cancer 21
 see also mastectomy

Calvinism 124, 143
cancer
 association with old age 23–5
 collective representations 22–3, 193
 consequences of symptoms 20
 and loss of independence 31–3
 narratives 173, 189, 193
 significance of symptoms 20, 28
 temporality 19, 27
 threat to bodily integrity 26–31
capitalism 99–104, 143
Catholics
 perceptions of Protestants 137
 social interdependence 136, 138
 see also Ballymacross
charismata 50
class
 relations of 101
 sense of membership 101
command, relations of 101
communicative interaction 88
competing knowledges 21
consciousness 60
consumerism 102, 118, 119
continuity, psychological 59–60, 190
conversion, religious 50
culture, post-modern 102, 103, 200

defeat 184–5
dementia 61, 64
 care in Eastern society 73
 loss of self in 68
 parent fixation in 70
 see also Alzheimer's disease

development, human 64
deviance
  primary 11
  secondary 11
diabetes 10
disabled identity 14
disease 4
doctors, role 11–12
drum making 142

empiricism 60
emplotment, therapeutic 173
epilepsy 13, 184–5
exercise
  distinguished from sport 106
  health benefits 105–6
  psychological health benefits 106
experiential coherence 187

feminist theory, and chronic illness 21
fitness industry 110
Foucault, M. 104

gay health professionals 153, 163–4
gay identity 149, 166–7
  and mental health 150–1, 166
gay men
  encounter with mental health
      professionals 152
  mental health 151–2
  population 149
  self-identity 149
  see also gay people's experiences in
      mental health services
gay people's experiences in mental
    health services 153–67
  conclusions 166–7
  data collection 153–4
  defensive language of clients 163–6
  heterosexism 157–61
  homophobia 156–7
  misattributions and stereotypes
      161–3
  positive encounters 154–6
gay subculture 149
gender roles 194–5
genetic identity 14
globalisation 99, 100, 201–2
'glocalisation' 100
glossolalia see speaking in tongues
governmentality 104, 119

Habermas, J. 88–9
habitus 101, 142
  class 101
  of Irish Catholics 125
  of rugby club 115–16
hair loss 26
Hall, S. 87–8
healing
  lay 134–5
  religious 53–4
  spiritual gift of 50
heteronormativity 152
heterosexism 152, 157–61
homophobia 152, 156–7
homosexuality
  incidence 149
  as mental pathology 150
human development 64
Hume, David 60
Hunterstown 130–2
  Catholics in 140–1, 144
  class issues 135–6
  religious denominations 131, 143
  restrictive ethos 144
  sub-divided community 141
  see also Northern Ireland health study

identity
  class 135
  collective 95
  concrete 61
  couple 69
  crisis of 102, 117–18
  development of concept 1–4
  disabled 14
  ethnicity and 83–6
  family influence 68–70
  formation of 101–2, 103, 118
  formed by experience 180
  gay see gay identity
  gendered 28–30, 194–5
  genetic 14
  and good health 178
  illness see illness identity
  linked to poor health in Irish 93–6
  maintenance work 70
  for marginalised 42–3
  meaning 59
  moral 191–3
  public 2
  religious see religious identity
  social see social identity

social psychological accounts 3–4
structures of 187–90
theories of 87–9
transformation of 38
transposable 103
see also narrative
illness 4
covering 13
as occupation 189
passing 13
illness career 15
illness experience 4–9
authenticity 5
illness identity 7
acceptance 14
image 61–2
impression management 62
independence, loss of 31–3
individualisation 102
individualism 62, 119, 200
individuality 59
injuries, sports 108–9
'inner loneliness' 144
interaction, symbolic 87
'interactive me' 3
introspection, sympathetic 2
IRA 82
Ireland, emigration from 78–81
'push' factors 79
see also Northern Ireland
Irish
experience in England 81–2
jokes 81–2
racialisation of 96
Irish in London
discrimination against 94–5
ethnicity and identity 83–6
health 90–2
identity and health links 93–6
study methodology 86–7
theories of identity 87–9

Jews in America 93

knowledges, competing 21
Korbut, Olga 107

labelling 11, 12
language 88–9
lay healing 134–5
lesbians

encounter with mental health
professionals 152
mental health 151–2
population 149
self-identity 149
see also gay people's experiences in
mental health services
life narratives *see* narrative
lifeworld 88–9
Lineker, Gary 108
liver disease 194
Locke, John 60, 61
loneliness 94
inner 144

madness 41–2
malignant mirroring 63
manliness 118
masculinity 13, 195
mastectomy 28–31
and ethnic community membership
30–1
and gendered identity 28–30
ME 177, 190
Mead, G.H. 87, 88
memory 59–60
episodic 60
false 60
as source of personal identity 60
meningitis 184–5
mental illness, and social identity 41–2
'metanarratives' 103
MIND 152
modernity 124
moral ethnographies 191
moral identities 191–3
motherhood 185–6
Myalism 41

narrative
broken 187
cancer 173, 189, 193
cause and effect in 192–3
chaos 171
contingent 172, 186
conventions 174–5
core 172, 179
genres 171–2
habitual 175
health and illness 176–86
method 21–2
moral 172, 174, 191–3

[narrative]
  observation sub-narrative 178
  past, present and future in 187–90
  progressive personal 171
  purposes 172–4, 194–5
  quest 171, 173
  regressive 171, 190
  research 175–6
  restitution 171
  of social identity 193–5
  stable 171
  themes in 186–7
nervousness 181–2
Northern Ireland 123–44
  health care research 126–8
  health concerns 126, 144
  health study in see Northern Ireland
    health study
  religious sectarianism 125
  social concerns 126
  unemployment 125, 129
Northern Ireland health study 128–44
  alcohol and diet 133
  background 128
  context 129–32
  discussion 142–4
  gender and health 133–4
  health beliefs 134–5
  religion, identity and health
    experiences 135–9
  religion, location and disadvantage
    140–1
  religion and risk 141
  rural health experiences 132–3
  social isolation and health 139–40

old age, societal view of 62–4
Orange Institution 131–2

PACE 152
parent fixation 70
Parfit, Derek 60
Pentecostalism 37–55
  community outreach 52
  continuity offered 40–1, 42
  critique of Western culture 55
  healing 53–4
  home cells 44–5
  identity for marginalised 42–3
  ontological belief 43–4
  speaking in tongues 42, 44, 50, 53
  spiritual gifts 50

spirituality 44, 50
spiritual walk 49
views on mental illness 45–8
worship 45, 50
personhood 59–61, 74
  'situated-embodied-agent' view 61
Pontypridd RFC 115–17
post-modernity 102, 103, 200
Post Natal Depression (PND) 139–40
primary deviance 11
'principle of compatibility' 102
private identity see self
prophecy 50
Protestants
  denominational divisions 131, 143
  independence/individuality 124, 143
  perceptions of Catholics 136
  see also Hunterstown
public identity 2
  see also social identity

racism 94–6
  institutionalised 95
rationalism 124
recognition, demand for 118–19
Reformation 124
relativism 55, 103
religion
  Calvinist 124, 143
  conflict with psychiatry 40, 54
  conversion 50
  as culture 125
  defining 123–4
  and health care 124–5
  and mental health 38
  see also Catholics; Northern Ireland
    health study; Pentecostalism;
    Protestants
religious identity 39, 48
  ethnic 125, 143, 144
  and mental health 39–40
rugby 108, 112–17
  career phases 113–14
  commodification of 116
  dealing with pain 116–17
  injury rates 108, 113
  physical preparation 114
  psychological preparation 115
rural accidents 141

sacred canopies 123
same sex attraction 149

Sartre, Jean-Paul 201
schizophrenia 54–5
Schwarzenegger, Arnold 111
secondary deviance 11
secularisation 143
self 2–3
   'ancestral' 60
   authentic selfhood 34
   'descendant' 60
   discontinuous 19, 25
   inter-subjective 33–4
   loss of 68, 190
   reflexive 87
   'Self One' 68
   'Self Three' 68
   'Self Two' 68, 69
   singular 68, 74
   technologies of 104, 110, 119
self-responsibility 184
self-understanding, through illness 6
sick role 6–7, 11–12
social capital 142–3, 144, 176
social constructionism 67
social identity 3, 193–5, 196
   and mental illness 41–2
   see also public identity
social standards, deviation from 10–11
speaking in tongues (glossolalia) 42, 44,
   50, 53
spirit possession 40–1, 46–8, 52–3

spirituality 44, 50
spiritual walk 49
spontaneity, loss of 10
sport
   bodybuilding 110–12
   competitiveness of 106–7
   and search for identity 117–19
   threat to health 107–9
   typology by health threat 109
   see also exercise; rugby
stigma, felt 14
stress 93–4, 179–80
subjectivism 143
'subjunctivising reality' 189
suffering
   as essential to human condition 6
   as redemptive 32–3
suicide 90, 93
survivorship 180–1
symbolic interaction 87
sympathetic introspection 2

technologies of the self 104, 110, 119
therapeutic emplotment 173

ulcerative colitis 9, 172

violence, as entertainment 119

wartime experience 180–1, 194